Ayurveda for Her

Practical Solutions to Strengthen Digestive System, Balance Hormones, Calm Stress and Embrace Natural Healing with Daily Self-Care Using Simple Ayurvedic Rituals

Isabella Harmony

© **Copyright 2025 by Isabella Harmony- All rights reserved.**

The content contained within this book may not be reproduced, duplicated, or transmitted without direct written permission from the author or the publisher. Under no circumstances will any blame or legal responsibility be held against the publisher or author for any damages, reparation, or monetary loss due to the information contained within this book, either directly or indirectly.

Legal Notice:

This book is copyright-protected. It is only for personal use. You cannot amend, distribute, sell, use, quote, or paraphrase any part of the content within this book without the consent of the author or publisher.

Disclaimer Notice:

Please note that the information contained within this document is for educational and entertainment purposes only. All efforts have been made to present accurate, up-to-date, and reliable, complete information. No warranties of any kind are declared or implied. Readers acknowledge that the author is not engaging in the rendering of legal, Financial, medical, or professional advice.

The content within this book has been derived from various sources. Please consult a licensed professional before attempting any techniques outlined in this book. By reading this document, the reader agrees that under no circumstances is the author responsible for any losses, direct or indirect, which are incurred as a result of the use of the information contained within this document, including but not limited to errors, omissions, or inaccuracies.

Table of Contents

Introduction 9

Chapter 1: Understanding Ayurvedic Foundations 11

    The Essence of Doshas: Vata, Pitta, and Kapha in Women 11

    Agni and Ama: Balancing Digestive Fire and Eliminating Toxins 13

    Dinacharya: Crafting a Daily Routine for Women's Well-being 14

    Prana and Ojas: Enhancing Vitality and Immunity Naturally.... 21

    Understanding Your Unique Constitution: A Personalized Approach 22

    Integrating Ayurveda with Modern Health Practices 24

Chapter 2: Holistic Hormonal Health 27

    Menstrual Health Reflection 28

    Natural Solutions for Hormonal Acne 29

    Acne Management Checklist 30

    Balancing Ayurveda with Hormonal Changes During Menopause 31

    Managing PMS with Ayurvedic Herbs and Diet 32

    PMS Symptom Tracker 34

    Supporting Thyroid Health through Ayurveda 34

    Nurturing Emotional Balance: Ayurvedic Practices for Mood Swings 36

Chapter 3: Digestive Wellness and Nutrition 39

    Dosha Meal Planning Checklist 40

    Recipes for Reducing Bloating and Indigestion 41

Mindful Eating Reflection Section 42
Seasonal Eating: Aligning Diet with Ayurvedic Seasons 42
Seasonal Eating Reflection Section 44
Mindful Eating: Cultivating a Sattvic Approach to Meals 44
Gratitude Practice for Meals 45
Kitchari Cleanses: A Gentle Detox for Women 46
Incorporating Superfoods: Turmeric, Ashwagandha, and More 48

Chapter 4: Life Stage Transitions and Ayurveda 51
Fertility and Ayurveda: Enhancing Reproductive Health 51
Emotional Well-Being Reflection Section 52
Pregnancy 52
Pregnancy Reflection Section 54
Postpartum Care: Rejuvenation and Recovery 54
Navigating Menopause Naturally with Ayurvedic Support 56
Menopause Reflection Section 57
Supporting Bone Health in Aging Women 58
Bone Health Checklist 59
Embracing the Wisdom Years: Ayurveda for Senior Women 59

Chapter 5: Spiritual and Cultural Integration 63
Personal Meditation Mantra 64
Understanding Chakras: Energy Centers and Women's Health 65
Chakra Health Checklist 66
Exploring Pranayama: Yogic Breathing for Stress Relief 67
Pranayama Practice Reflection 68
Cultivating Mindfulness: Integrating Ayurveda into Daily Life .. 69

Cultural Sensitivity: Respectful Practice of Ayurveda 70

Personal Empowerment through Ayurvedic Rituals 73

Exploring Your Intentions 74

Chapter 6: Practical Self-Care Strategies 75

Self-Care Toolkit Checklist 76

Ayurvedic Skin Care: Natural Beauty Practices 77

Ayurvedic Skincare Routine Checklist 78

Sleep and Ayurveda: Enhancing Restorative Sleep Naturally .. 78

Stress Management: Ayurvedic Techniques for Calmness 80

Stress Management Reflection Exercise 81

Building Resilience: Strengthening Immunity with Ayurveda ... 82

Ayurvedic Aromatherapy: Using Essential Oils for Healing 83

Chapter 7: Overcoming Common Objections and Misconceptions 87

Demystifying Ayurvedic Complexity: Simple Practices for Beginners 87

Time-Efficient Ayurveda: Integrating Practices into a Busy Schedule 88

Cost-Effective Ayurveda: Affordable Solutions for Every Budget 90

Navigating Skepticism: Evidence-Based Benefits of Ayurveda 92

Ayurveda and Western Medicine: Finding a Harmonious Balance 94

Chapter 8: Personal Stories and Transformative Journeys 97

From Burnout to Balance: A Journey of Healing and Renewal . 97

Balance and Renewal Checklist 98

Overcoming Digestive Struggles 99

Digestive Health Reflection Exercise 100

Hormonal Harmony: Personal Triumphs with Ayurveda........ 100

Hormonal Health Reflection Section 102

Embracing Self-Care 102

Self-Care Reflection Journal 104

Cultural Connection: Finding Identity through Ayurveda 104

Cultural Reflection and Integration Journal 106

Transformative Change: The Path to Holistic Health and Well-being... 106

Chapter 9: Eat Well, Feel Well: Simple Ayurvedic Recipes 109

Ayurvedic Kitchen Essentials: Stock Your Ayurvedic Pantry .. 109

Recipes: 110

Cucumber & Dill Cooling Salad 110

Spiced Yogurt with Cumin 111

Simple Lentil Digestive Soup 112

Stewed Apples with Cinnamon 113

Quinoa with Ginger & Veggies 114

Digestive Herbal Blend Tea (CCFG) 115

Tea & Tonic Recipes 116

Warm Spiced Oatmeal (Vata-balancing breakfast) 117

Kitchari Power Bowl (Balanced doshas, easy digestion) 118

Quinoa & Veggie Power Salad *(Ideal for Kapha-balance)* 119

Spiced Sweet Potato & Chickpea Snack *(Balanced afternoon pick-me-up)* 120

Warm Cardamom Pear Stew (Evening dessert or snack) 121

Serves 2 121

Menstrual Ease Moong-Pear Stew 122

Balancing Evening Golden Milk 123

Hormone-Balancing Chia & Oat Breakfast Bowl 124

PMS Ease Seed Cycling Smoothie 125

Seasonal Spring Mung & Asparagus Khichdi........................ 126

Hormone-Balancing Seed & Date Bars 127

Tridoshic Energy Balls 128

Calming Ashwagandha-Almond Bites 129

Spring (Kapha Season) 130

Summer (Pitta Season) 131

Autumn (Early Vata Season).. 132

Winter (Deep Vata Season) 133

Conclusion 137

References 139

Introduction

In the heart of a fast-paced, noisy city, Anjali began to notice something was off. Her energy had dipped, her sleep had become restless, and a quiet, persistent unease followed her through the day. Life felt out of balance. One afternoon, during a conversation with her grandmother, a familiar word resurfaced: Ayurveda. She had heard it before but never truly listened. This time, it sparked something. What began as a search for relief became a deeper journey—one that reconnected her with her roots and introduced her to a way of living that brought calm, clarity, and a renewed sense of self.

The same journey inspires Ayurveda for Her - one of curiosity, discovery, and healing. It's written for the modern woman navigating the pressures of daily life, offering practical, down-to-earth ways to care for her health using the timeless wisdom of Ayurveda. But this book is more than just wellness tips. It's an invitation to return to yourself, to find balance in your body, mind, and spirit.

My path to Ayurveda began years ago, fueled by a deep interest in natural wellness and a desire to understand what truly supports long-term health. Along the way, I explored Ayurvedic practices in my own life, drawing from a blend of trusted resources, research, and real-world application. The changes I experienced were powerful, and I've seen similar transformations in the lives of many other women as well. This book is a reflection of that lived experience—one I hope will empower and inspire you.

Whether you're a young woman trying to find your rhythm in a fast-paced world, a mother giving so much of yourself to others, or someone entering a new season of life seeking clarity and renewal, this book was created with you in mind. You'll find guidance to support your digestion, balance hormones, improve sleep, and nurture your emotional well-being. These aren't abstract theories; they're practical steps you can gently fold into your day.

This journey is about transformation, not perfection. Even small shifts can lead to powerful changes. Ayurveda reminds us that when we live in tune with ourselves, we unlock a deeper vitality and peace that no external fix can provide.

So, as you read these pages, I invite you to be kind to yourself. Let this be a supportive companion on your wellness path. Allow the practices to meet you where you are. May this book bring you closer to feeling vibrant, steady, and whole, and help you reconnect with the wisdom that's always been within you.

Chapter 1: Understanding Ayurvedic Foundations

You find yourself amid daily chaos, work deadlines, family responsibilities, and the constant pull of social obligations. It becomes easy to forget the importance of nurturing yourself. In the whirlwind, you might notice subtle cues: a restless mind, a disconnected body, skin that doesn't glow like it used to. These are the whispers of imbalance, gently nudging you to listen. Ayurveda, an ancient practice from India, offers a way back to harmony. It invites you to understand your body's unique needs, guiding you toward a state of equilibrium. Let's explore how the wisdom of the doshas can illuminate your path to well-being, offering timeless yet relevant insights that are truly valuable.

The Essence of Doshas: Vata, Pitta, and Kapha in Women

At the heart of Ayurveda lies the concept of doshas. These energies govern our physiological and psychological functions and are as unique to us as our fingerprints. Understanding your dosha is like having a compass for your health. Vata, Pitta, and Kapha are the three primary doshas, each playing a vital role in shaping who you are.

Vata, composed of air and space, is the dosha of movement and creativity. Women with a dominant Vata constitution tend to be light and airy, both physically and mentally. You might be quick to think and express yourself, but just as fast to feel anxious or overwhelmed. Dry skin, irregular digestion, and restlessness are familiar companions when Vata is out of balance.

Then there's Pitta, the fiery dosha, ruled by the elements of fire and water. If Pitta is your dominant dosha, you likely possess intensity and determination. You're driven, with a sharp intellect. But that fire can sometimes burn too brightly, leading to inflammation, irritability, or impatience. When Pitta becomes out of balance, you may notice skin rashes, digestive issues, or even episodes of anger.

Kapha, the dosha of earth and water, embodies stability and strength. With Kapha as your guiding force, you may find yourself grounded and have a steady disposition. People often describe you as nurturing and compassionate. However, excess Kapha can lead to sluggishness, weight gain, and a feeling of being stuck. You may struggle with lethargy or find it difficult to let go of things.

Recognizing which dosha is predominant in your constitution is a powerful first step. There are various ways to identify your dosha. Self-assessment quizzes are a great start, prompting you to reflect on your physical traits and emotional tendencies. You may also want to observe your preferences and daily habits. Do you crave spicy foods or cool environments? Are you drawn to rigorous workouts or gentle strolls?

Once you understand your dosha, the next step is balancing it. If Vata is your dominant dosha, incorporating grounding practices can be beneficial. Warm, cooked foods, regular sleep schedules, and calming practices such as yoga or meditation can help soothe an overactive mind. For Pitta, cooling foods such as cucumbers and melons, along with stress management techniques, can help temper your inner fire. Practicing mindfulness and spending time in nature can also be beneficial. If Kapha is your guide, focus on stimulating activities that keep you moving, such as brisk walks or invigorating workouts. Opt for light, spicy meals and ensure you stay engaged with new experiences.

Finding your balance is not about changing who you are; it's about discovering who you are. It's about honoring your natural tendencies while gently guiding them toward a state of harmony. Ayurveda teaches us that health is dynamic, a dance of the doshas. By understanding and nurturing your unique constitution, you can cultivate a life that not only feels good but is also deeply fulfilling.

Agni and Ama: Balancing Digestive Fire and Eliminating Toxins

In the realm of Ayurveda, your well-being is intricately linked to the balance of Agni, the digestive fire, and the elimination of Ama, toxins that cloud the body and mind. Think of Agni as the flame that powers your body's engine. It is the force that digests food, assimilates nutrients, and fuels your vitality. A strong Agni is a beacon of health; it ensures that your body efficiently transforms food into energy, leaving you feeling vibrant and alive. However, when Agni is weak, digestion falters, and undigested food becomes Ama. This toxic sludge has a profound impact on health, manifesting as fatigue, persistent digestive issues, and a general sense of heaviness.

Ama forms when digestion is impaired, often due to poor eating habits, stress, or an unhealthy lifestyle. Picture a sluggish river, clogged with debris; this is how Ama stagnates within, blocking the flow of nutrients and energy. Women, in particular, may notice symptoms such as bloating, dull skin, or a foggy mind when Ama takes hold. It is as if the body sends subtle distress signals, urging you to clear the clutter and reignite the digestive flame. The journey to reclaiming your health begins by tending to Agni and reducing the toxic load of Ama.

Consider incorporating warming spices like ginger and cumin into your meals to nourish Agni. These spices act as kindling, stoking the digestive fire and enhancing your body's ability to break down food. Mindful eating, a simple yet profound practice, is crucial. By savoring each bite and avoiding distractions like screens and multitasking, you allow your body to engage fully in the digestion process. It is an invitation to slow down, to be present, and to honor the nourishment before you.

Detoxification is another cornerstone of Ayurveda, a practice that aligns with your body's natural rhythms and seasons. Gentle detox routines, such as sipping herbal teas or engaging in intermittent fasting, can help eliminate Ama. These practices are not about deprivation but about creating space for rejuvenation. Seasonal cleansing, tailored to the body's needs during different times of the year, supports this process. For instance, spring, with its renewing energy, is an ideal time for detox. A simple cleanse may involve consuming lighter foods, such as soups and salads, reducing heavy and processed foods, and incorporating practices like dry brushing to stimulate lymphatic drainage.

Incorporating these Ayurvedic practices into daily life does not require dramatic overhauls. It's about making small, meaningful changes that resonate with your lifestyle. Imagine starting your day with a cup of warm ginger tea, setting the tone for a balanced digestive system. Or take a few moments before meals to breathe deeply and express gratitude for your food. These seemingly small moments can create ripples of well-being throughout your life.

Ayurveda teaches that health is a dynamic equilibrium. By nurturing Agni and reducing Ama, you cultivate a body that is not only free from disease but is a vessel of vitality and joy. This ancient wisdom offers a roadmap to understanding your body's unique needs, inviting you to listen, to nurture, and to thrive. As you explore these practices, you may find yourself more attuned to your body's whispers and more empowered in your health journey.

Dinacharya: Crafting a Daily Routine for Women's Well-being

Imagine waking up each morning with a profound sense of purpose and direction, your day unfolding with an elegant, natural rhythm that feels both intensely productive and genuinely nurturing to your soul. This is the transformative promise of Dinacharya, the ancient Ayurvedic concept of a daily routine that thoughtfully aligns your activities with the natural cycles of the day and the subtle energies that govern our world. More than simply a schedule to follow, Dinacharya represents a sacred dance between your inner rhythms and the external world, honoring the wisdom that our ancestors understood—that we are intimately connected to the patterns of nature, from the rising and setting of the sun to the seasonal changes that influence our physical, mental, and emotional well-being.

In Ayurveda, consistency emerges as the fundamental cornerstone of vibrant health and lasting vitality. This isn't about rigidity or perfection, but rather about creating a gentle, sustainable framework that supports your body's natural intelligence. Establishing a well-crafted routine serves as powerful medicine, systematically balancing the three doshas—Vata (the energies of movement and change), Pitta (the forces of transformation and metabolism), and Kapha (the principles of structure and stability), while simultaneously strengthening your body's innate resilience and adaptive capacity. As you embrace this structured daily rhythm with patience and dedication, you may notice remarkable transformations: sustained energy that carries you through your day without the peaks and crashes of modern living, enhanced mental clarity and focus that allows you to approach challenges with grace, improved digestive function that leaves you feeling light and nourished, better sleep quality that truly restores your body and mind, and an overall greater sense of well-being that radiates from within and touches every aspect of your life. Dinacharya transcends the boundaries of a mere routine; it becomes a transformative way of life that actively fosters harmony between your deepest needs and the demands of daily existence.

Begin your day with intentional morning rituals that consciously set the tone for balance, vitality, and inner peace throughout the hours ahead. The ancient practice of rising early, ideally in the magical window between 5:30 and 6:00 AM, before the sun rises, allows you to capture the pristine, peaceful energy of dawn time when the world is naturally quiet and your mind is most receptive to stillness and intention. This early rising isn't about forcing yourself awake, but rather about gradually training your body to align with nature's rhythm, creating space for yourself before the world awakens with its endless demands and distractions.

Engage in time-honored practices like tongue scraping, using a simple copper or stainless-steel tool to gently remove the toxins and bacteria that have accumulated overnight as your body processes the previous day's experiences and emotions. This ancient practice, validated by modern research, not only improves oral health but also stimulates the organs and awakens your digestive system for the day ahead. Follow this with oil pulling, a deep cleansing practice where you swish a tablespoon of sesame or coconut oil in your mouth for 10-15 minutes while you prepare for your day, effectively removing harmful bacteria, improving gum health, and even supporting clearer skin and fresher breath. These simple actions, rooted in thousands of years of wisdom and understanding of the body's natural detoxification processes, prepare your entire system to greet the day with a clean slate, both physically and energetically.

As you move through your morning routine with mindfulness and intention, consider incorporating precious minutes of meditation or gentle yoga, allowing your mind to settle into its natural state of calm and clarity before the day's inevitable demands take hold. This might be as simple as five minutes of deep breathing while you drink your first glass of warm water, or a more extended practice of gentle stretches and sun salutations that honor your body and the new day. These sacred rituals serve as your daily anchor, grounding you in the present moment and offering a consistent foundation of peace and intentionality that you can return to throughout even the most challenging days.

As the sun reaches its powerful zenith and the day's energy peaks, shift your focus to midday practices that skillfully sustain your energy and support your body's natural rhythms. This is the time when your digestive fire burns strongest, making it the ideal window for your most substantial meal of the day. Make time for a truly mindful meal, creating a sanctuary of nourishment by removing distractions like phones, computers, or television, and instead savoring each bite with complete attention and gratitude for the earth's abundance. This practice of mindful eating not only significantly aids digestion by allowing your body to recognize and properly process the food you're consuming but also creates a moment of meditation within your day, enabling you to appreciate the colors, textures, flavors, and life-giving properties of your nourishment.

Consider taking a moment to step outside after lunch, even if only for a few precious moments of connection with nature. The midday sun provides essential vitamin D, which supports bone health, immune function, and mood regulation. Meanwhile, fresh air invigorates the spirit and offers a natural boost to both mood and mental focus through the simple act of breathing deeply and consciously. This midday pause becomes more than just a break; it's an opportunity to reset your entire system, ensuring that the afternoon is met with renewed vigor, sustained energy, and clear focus rather than the post-meal fatigue that so many experience in our modern, indoor-focused lifestyle.

As evening gracefully approaches and the day's activities begin to wind down, craft a nurturing routine that gently guides your body and mind from activity toward rest, honoring the natural transition from day to night. Engage in naturally calming activities that signal to your nervous system that it's time to release the day's tensions and prepare for restoration. This might include reading inspiring books that feed your soul, listening to soothing music or nature sounds that calm your mind, practicing gentle stretches that release physical tension from your body, or engaging in creative activities like journaling, drawing, or crafts that bring you joy without overstimulation.

An early bedtime, ideally by 10 p.m., aligns perfectly with your body's natural circadian rhythms and takes advantage of the naturally drowsy period that occurs as Kapha energy increases in the evening hours. This isn't about depriving yourself of evening activities, but rather about recognizing that quality sleep is one of the most potent medicines available to you, supporting everything from immune function and emotional regulation to mental clarity and physical repair. Consider incorporating rituals that signal to your entire being that it's time for rest: a warm bath infused with Epsom salts and calming essential oils like lavender or chamomile, which not only relax your muscles but also provide aromatherapy benefits that calm your nervous system, or sipping a cup of herbal tea, perhaps chamomile for its gentle sedative properties, passionflower for nervous system support, or a traditional Ayurvedic blend specifically designed to promote deep, restorative sleep.

This evening routine becomes your sanctuary, creating a consistent bridge between the active energy of the day and the restorative embrace of night, preparing you for the kind of deep, rejuvenating sleep that allows you to wake naturally refreshed and ready to embrace a new day with enthusiasm and vitality.

Personalizing Dinacharya to honor and support your unique needs, constitution, and life circumstances is essential to its long-term success and sustainability. The beauty of Ayurvedic wisdom lies in its recognition that there is no one-size-fits-all approach to health and well-being. Adapting routines for different doshas ensures that each practice genuinely supports your individual constitution while addressing any current imbalances in your body, mind, or emotions.

For instance, if you tend toward Vata characteristics, you may be naturally creative, energetic, and changeable, but also prone to anxiety, irregular digestion, or difficulty with routine. In such cases, you might benefit tremendously from grounding activities that provide stability and warmth. This could include consistent meal times with nourishing, cooked foods, regular oil massage to calm the nervous system, gentle and consistent exercise such as walking or restorative yoga, and creating warm, nurturing environments in your home and workspace.

Those with predominantly Pitta qualities may be naturally focused, ambitious, and intelligent, but also prone to irritability, inflammation, or burnout. They might find balance through cooling practices and creating space for downtime. This could involve favoring cooling foods and drinks, scheduling regular periods of rest and relaxation, practicing cooling breathing techniques, and ensuring your environment isn't overly heated or stimulating.

If Kapha tendencies dominate your constitution, you may be naturally calm, stable, and nurturing, but also prone to sluggishness, weight gain, or resistance to change. In such cases, you might thrive with more stimulating and energizing practices. This could include waking earlier to avoid oversleeping, incorporating more vigorous movement and exercise, choosing lighter, warming foods and spices, and engaging in activities that challenge and invigorate you.

Life stages also profoundly influence your optimal routine, and Ayurveda honors these natural transitions with great wisdom. During pregnancy, your body and spirit require extra nurturing and rest, accompanied by gentle practices that support both you and your growing baby. During menopause, cooling and calming activities might help ease the intensity of this powerful transition, while practices that honor your accumulated wisdom become especially important. Young mothers might need to adapt their routines to shorter, more flexible practices that can be maintained despite the beautiful chaos of caring for small children.

Consistency emerges as the absolute foundation of any successful and transformative routine, but this doesn't mean perfection or rigidity. The ancient texts remind us that even small practices performed with love and dedication over time can create profound and lasting changes in our lives, while sporadic, intense efforts often lead to burnout and abandonment of the very practices that could support us the most.

Setting gentle reminders and creating supportive systems can help maintain your commitment to Dinacharya without adding stress to your life. You might make a beautiful daily checklist that feels inspiring rather than overwhelming, set gentle phone alarms with meaningful messages that remind you of your intentions, or place visual cues around your home that connect you to the deeper purpose behind your practices. Sharing your routine with a trusted friend or family member can provide invaluable support and encouragement, creating a sense of loving accountability that motivates rather than judges.

The key is to integrate these practices into your life in a way that feels natural, sustainable, and genuinely nourishing rather than like another item on your endless to-do list. Start small, with just one or two practices that resonate most deeply with your heart and current needs, and gradually build your routine over weeks and months, allowing each new habit to become woven into the fabric of your life before adding the next.

Dinacharya is not about rigid adherence to a predetermined schedule or forcing yourself into a lifestyle that doesn't honor your unique circumstances. Instead, it's about discovering a natural, flowing rhythm that harmoniously integrates with your life's demands, responsibilities, and deepest aspirations. It offers a time-tested path to sustainable balance, where the inevitable chaos and unpredictability of the external world are met with the grounded calm and intentional presence that comes from a life lived in alignment with natural wisdom.

Prana and Ojas: Enhancing Vitality and Immunity Naturally

Prana, the life force that flows within us, animating our bodies and minds. In Ayurveda, Prana is not merely breath but the energy that sustains life itself, coursing through every cell. It fuels your creativity, powers your movement, and ignites your spirit. When Prana flows freely, you feel alive and connected. On the other hand, Ojas is the sap of life, the vital essence that fortifies your immunity and resilience. It is the nectar of health, providing strength and vitality. Prana and Ojas form the foundation of well-being, ensuring you thrive in body, mind, and spirit.

To cultivate Prana and Ojas, consider incorporating simple practices into your life. Breathing exercises, like Pranayama, enhance the flow of Prana. Deep, conscious breathing calms the nervous system and increases oxygen intake, invigorating your body and clearing your mind. Nourishment also plays a crucial role. Foods like ghee and almonds are rich in nutrients that build Ojas, supporting your immune system and vitality. Embrace restorative activities like yoga and meditation, which harmonize Prana and nurture Ojas, leaving you centered and refreshed. These practices are not mere tasks but opportunities to replenish your life force, making every moment a chance to renew and recharge.

Protecting Prana and Ojas from depletion is essential, especially in a world of distractions and demands. Consider how lifestyle choices impact these vital forces. Overstimulation, such as excessive screen time, can scatter Prana, leaving you feeling drained and unfocused. Prioritizing rest is vital for safeguarding Ojas. Quality sleep is the body's natural way of restoring balance, allowing Prana to flow and Ojas to rebuild. Create a sanctuary for rest by establishing a calming bedtime routine free from digital distractions. Your body will thank you with increased vitality and a fortified immune system. It's about creating boundaries that honor your energy and preserve your essence.

Emotional well-being is intricately linked to Prana and Ojas. Emotions, like waves, ebb and flow, impacting your energy and vitality. Cultivating emotional balance is crucial for sustaining Prana and nurturing Ojas. Journaling can be a powerful practice, offering a space to express and process emotions, freeing the mind, and invigorating the spirit. Gratitude exercises, where you reflect on the positive aspects of your life, shift your focus from scarcity to abundance, thereby enhancing emotional resilience. These practices foster a positive mindset, which is the soil in which Prana and Ojas flourish. A healthy emotional landscape supports a vibrant life force, enabling you to navigate life with grace and strength.

In the fast-paced rhythm of modern life, it is easy to overlook the subtle energies that sustain us. Yet, by tuning into Prana and Ojas, you can create a life that not only survives but also thrives. These concepts, though ancient, offer timeless wisdom for nurturing vitality and fostering resilience. Integrating breathing exercises, nourishing foods, restorative activities, and emotional practices builds a reservoir of vitality that supports every aspect of your life. This holistic approach to health invites you to listen, nurture, and flourish, recognizing your innate potential for well-being.

Understanding Your Unique Constitution: A Personalized Approach

Each one of us is unique yet connected by the shared experience of being human. Just like fingerprints, each of us has a distinct Ayurvedic constitution that shapes our health and well-being. In Ayurveda, recognizing this individuality is crucial. No single diet or lifestyle suits all, and this ancient wisdom teaches us to honor our differences. It's about crafting a personal map that guides you toward balance, allowing you to thrive in your own skin. This approach is liberating, freeing you from the one-size-fits-all mentality of modern health trends.

Determining your unique Ayurvedic constitution, known as Prakriti, is the first step in understanding your health. This involves understanding the balance of the three doshas —Vata, Pitta, and Kapha —within you. A handy tool for this self-discovery is the constitution quiz. These quizzes prompt you to reflect on your physical characteristics, emotional tendencies, and lifestyle preferences. Perhaps you have a slender frame, a quick mind, and a love for spontaneous adventures. These traits might indicate a Vata dominance. Or maybe you have a strong build, a fiery temperament, and a penchant for leadership, which suggests a Pitta constitution. Kapha might be your guiding force if you're more grounded, with a calm demeanor and a love for routine. Observing your habits and preferences can also offer insights. Professional consultations with Ayurvedic practitioners provide deeper guidance, offering personalized insights and recommendations based on a detailed assessment.

Once you understand your constitution, you can tailor your health practices to support balance and overall well-being. Diet is a powerful tool in this personalization process. Consider Pitta types, who may thrive on cooling foods like cucumber and melon to temper their inner fire, while Vata types benefit from warm, nourishing meals like soups and stews. Kapha individuals may find that lighter meals with a hint of spice help maintain their energy levels. Lifestyle adjustments are equally necessary. If you're a Vata type, grounding activities like yoga can help calm your busy mind. Pittas might benefit from stress-reducing practices like meditation, while Kaphas stay energized with stimulating exercises like brisk walking.

This personalized approach extends beyond diet and exercise. It invites you to explore the mind-body connection, integrating practices that nurture your spirit. Meditation and yoga are powerful allies in this quest, fostering mindfulness and inner peace. They help you tune into your body's rhythms and respond with kindness and care. Spiritual well-being is another key facet of holistic health. Incorporating mindfulness into daily life, through simple practices such as focused breathing or gratitude journaling, can enhance your sense of connection and fulfillment.

Ayurveda promotes a holistic perspective on health and wellness, where the mind, body, and spirit are inextricably intertwined. It invites you to look beyond symptoms and quick fixes, urging you to consider the whole person. This transformative perspective offers a path to true well-being that honors your unique essence. As you adopt this personalized approach, you may find yourself more attuned to your body's signals, more empowered in your health decisions, and more connected to the world around you.

In this way, Ayurveda offers a framework for understanding and nurturing your unique constitution, guiding you toward a life of balance and vitality. It's an invitation to explore and experiment, find what resonates with you, and integrate practices supporting your journey to holistic health.

Integrating Ayurveda with Modern Health Practices

In today's world, we often find ourselves at the crossroads of ancient traditions and modern healthcare. With its rich history, Ayurveda stands ready to complement contemporary medical practices. This integration can create a harmonious balance where both systems work together to enhance your health. Imagine having the best of both worlds: the wisdom of Ayurveda guiding you to support your body naturally while modern medicine provides precision and technology when needed. It's about choosing a path where these approaches coexist, enhancing your well-being with a comprehensive perspective. This isn't about replacing one with the other but finding synergy between them.

Integrative health combines Ayurveda with Western medicine seamlessly. For instance, while Western medicine might offer a quick fix for acute conditions, Ayurveda can provide long-term lifestyle adjustments to prevent recurrence. Think about the balance of a nutritious diet. By bringing Ayurvedic principles into modern nutrition, you can enjoy a diet that's not only balanced but also personalized. This might include swapping processed snacks for Ayurvedic superfoods like turmeric and amla or incorporating mindful eating practices to enhance digestion. These small changes can make a significant difference, blending traditional wisdom with current dietary standards.

Exercise is another area where fusion thrives. Combining yoga with other fitness practices can offer a holistic approach to physical well-being. Yoga provides flexibility, balance, and mental clarity, whereas a contemporary routine may focus on cardiovascular health or strength training. Together, they create a well-rounded exercise regimen that nourishes both the body and mind. Try out a week where you enjoy a gentle yoga class on Monday, a brisk walk on Wednesday, and a strength session on Friday. This balance ensures you address all aspects of fitness, staying active and engaged without burnout.

Misconceptions often cloud the understanding of Ayurveda in relation to modern medicine. Some may view Ayurveda as unscientific or outdated. However, evidence supports many Ayurvedic practices, highlighting their effectiveness and safety. For example, studies show the benefits of turmeric in reducing inflammation and supporting joint health. These findings bridge the gap between skepticism and evidence, demonstrating how Ayurveda can complement modern medicine. It's time to dispel myths and embrace the possibilities, recognizing that both systems have their strengths and can work together to achieve a healthier life.

Holistic wellness encompasses the concept of integrating mind, body, and spirit. This comprehensive view acknowledges that proper health involves more than just the absence of disease. It's about nurturing every aspect of your being. Ayurveda and modern practices can coexist harmoniously, offering a personalized health journey that encourages exploration and adaptation. Whether it's through meditation, dietary adjustments, or a combination of therapies, this holistic approach fosters a deep connection to yourself and the world around you.

Chapter 2: Holistic Hormonal Health

A woman's menstrual cycle is an essential indicator of her overall health. According to Ayurveda, menstruation is more than just a biological function; it reflects the body's internal balance and harmony. A regular, pain-free cycle is seen as a sign that the body and mind are in a state of harmony. When the cycle becomes irregular or uncomfortable, it may signal that something in the body needs attention or support.

The menstrual cycle in Ayurveda is divided into three phases: Vata, Pitta, and Kapha, each with distinct characteristics. The Vata phase, which encompasses menstruation itself, is a time of movement and release. During this time, you might feel more introspective or notice heightened sensitivity. Ensuring warmth and comfort can soothe the often-overactive Vata dosha. The body's transformative energy peaks as you transition into the Pitta phase, which typically occurs during ovulation. You might experience heightened creativity and motivation, yet managing this fiery energy is crucial to prevent imbalance. Finally, the Kapha phase leads to the premenstrual period, a time of building and preparation. Here, nourishing practices can help alleviate the heaviness and stagnation that may arise.

Imbalances within these phases often manifest as irregular cycles or painful periods, known as dysmenorrhea. For some, the cycle might even cease, a condition called amenorrhea. Ayurveda offers gentle yet effective remedies. Herbs like Ashoka and Shatavari are revered for their ability to harmonize and support menstrual health. Ashoka, known for its cooling properties, helps alleviate discomfort and regulate flow, while Shatavari nourishes and balances, addressing hormonal fluctuations. Alongside herbal support, lifestyle adjustments can provide relief. Yoga poses specifically targeting menstrual health, such as the reclining bound angle pose or gentle twists, can offer comfort and ease tension.

Diet plays an invaluable role in supporting menstrual health. By aligning your diet with the phases of the cycle, you can nourish your body in harmony with its natural rhythms. During the Vata phase, consider warm, grounding foods like soups and stews, which provide comfort and stability. As you move into the Pitta phase, cooling salads and hydrating fruits help balance the body's heat. In the Kapha phase, focus on light, energizing meals to counteract any sluggishness. Hydration is equally essential. Herbal teas, such as those infused with ginger or fennel, offer warmth, support digestion, and balance the doshas during menstruation.

Rest and relaxation are not mere indulgences but necessities during menstruation. In our fast-paced world, it's easy to overlook the importance of taking a moment to pause and reflect. However, your body craves rest, seeking time to rejuvenate and heal. Embrace restorative practices that encourage relaxation. Guided meditations can calm the mind, while gentle stretching releases tension from the body. With scents like lavender or chamomile, aromatherapy offers tranquility and can ease emotional fluctuations. Journaling provides a space for reflection, allowing you to connect with your inner self and express emotions that might surface during this time.

Menstrual Health Reflection

Take a moment to reflect on your menstrual cycle. Consider how you feel during each phase, emotionally, physically, and energetically. Are there patterns you notice? Use this space to jot down any observations or insights. This reflection is a step towards understanding and honoring your body's natural rhythms, offering a deeper connection to your menstrual health.

As you navigate the intricacies of hormonal health, remember that Ayurveda offers a lens through which you can view your cycle not as a burden but as a powerful indicator of your overall well-being. It invites you to listen to your body, nurture it with care, and embrace its wisdom. In doing so, you cultivate a deeper connection with yourself, fostering a sense of balance and harmony that resonates throughout every aspect of your life.

Natural Solutions for Hormonal Acne

Hormonal acne often feels like a persistent visitor, popping up at the most inconvenient times. From an Ayurvedic perspective, this condition is deeply tied to the balance of doshas in your body, particularly the Pitta dosha. When Pitta, the dosha associated with heat and transformation, becomes imbalanced, it can manifest as inflammation and heat on your skin, leading to those unwelcome breakouts. This imbalance might be triggered by stress, diet, or lifestyle choices, and understanding these triggers can be the first step in addressing the root cause of acne rather than just the symptoms.

Ayurveda offers a treasure trove of natural remedies that help manage hormonal acne while promoting overall skin health. Consider herbal face packs made from neem and turmeric. Neem, known for its antibacterial properties, helps clear up acne-causing bacteria, while turmeric acts as an anti-inflammatory powerhouse, reducing redness and swelling. Consider internal remedies like Triphala and aloe vera juice for more thorough cleansing. Triphala, a traditional herbal blend, aids digestion and detoxification, clearing internal toxins that might otherwise surface as skin issues. Aloe vera juice, with its cooling properties, helps soothe the digestive tract, supporting Pitta balance and encouraging clearer skin from the inside out.

Diet is another crucial factor in achieving radiant skin. Embrace anti-inflammatory foods, such as leafy greens and berries, which support your skin and benefit your overall health. These foods help reduce inflammation and provide essential nutrients that nourish your skin from the inside. On the flip side, avoid spicy and oily foods, which can exacerbate Pitta and lead to breakouts. By making mindful dietary choices, you support your body's natural healing processes and create an environment that allows your skin to thrive.

Stress often plays a significant role in the condition of your skin. Managing stress through lifestyle changes can significantly improve the control of acne. Incorporate stress-reduction techniques like breathing exercises and mindfulness practices into your daily routine. These practices help calm your mind and body, reducing the stress that can lead to Pitta imbalances. Additionally, consider refining your skincare routine with gentle cleansing and natural moisturizers. Opt for products that are free from harsh chemicals and artificial fragrances, as these can irritate your skin and exacerbate acne. A simple routine with natural products can help nurture your skin and maintain its balance.

Acne Management Checklist

To help you on your path to clearer skin, consider creating a checklist that includes daily practices and dietary guidelines. This checklist may include items such as drinking plenty of water, enjoying daily herbal tea, and setting aside time for stress-reducing activities. This tool gently reminds you of the small steps you can take daily to support your skin's health.

Hormonal acne can feel frustrating, but with Ayurveda, you have a compassionate ally. By addressing the root causes through natural remedies, thoughtful diet, and mindful lifestyle changes, you nurture your skin and your entire being. Embrace these practices and watch your skin reflect the inner balance and harmony you cultivate.

Balancing Ayurveda with Hormonal Changes During Menopause

Menopause, from an Ayurvedic perspective, isn't just an end but a natural transitional shift into a new phase of life. It's a time when the body naturally moves from a Pitta-driven phase of life to a Vata-dominant stage. This transition often brings changes, such as increased dryness, which can manifest in the skin and joints and can also stir feelings of anxiety. Ayurveda views this shift as a natural process and offers gentle ways to ease the accompanying symptoms. By understanding this transition as a rebalancing of doshas, you can approach menopause with a sense of empowerment and acceptance.

To manage these changes, Ayurveda suggests various strategies that work in harmony with your body. Herbal support can play a significant role in this process. Black cohosh and licorice are often recommended for their balancing properties. Black cohosh helps to alleviate hot flashes and night sweats, while licorice supports adrenal health, which can be particularly beneficial during this phase. Alongside herbal remedies, incorporating lifestyle practices such as regular exercise and meditation can be transformative. Gentle activities like walking or yoga not only keep the body flexible but also help maintain emotional equilibrium. Meditation offers a sanctuary for the mind, calming the storm of thoughts that can accompany hormonal shifts.

Diet is another cornerstone of navigating menopause with grace. Nourishing Vata through diet is key to maintaining balance. Warm, cooked meals that include healthy fats such as ghee and coconut oil, provide the body with grounding and nourishment. These foods counteract the drying nature of Vata, promoting moisture and vitality. On the other hand, it's wise to avoid cold and raw foods, which can aggravate Vata, leading to imbalances. Instead, think of hearty stews and soups that comfort both body and spirit, offering warmth and stability.

The emotional and mental well-being during menopause cannot be overstated. Hormonal changes can lead to mood swings and emotional upheavals and addressing these is just as vital as managing physical symptoms. Emotional support through counseling or support groups can offer a space to share experiences and feelings, providing a sense of community and understanding. Mindfulness practices like journaling and gratitude exercises allow for reflection and emotional processing. Writing down thoughts and feelings can be cathartic, helping to navigate the emotional landscape of menopause with clarity and calm.

Menopause is a unique time marked by significant changes and new beginnings in a woman's life. You can support your body and mind through this transition by embracing Ayurvedic practices. Ayurveda offers a holistic approach that sees menopause not as a loss but as an opportunity for growth and transformation. Through herbal support, mindful lifestyle choices, nourishing foods, and emotional care, you provide yourself with the tools to navigate this stage with wisdom and grace, honoring the natural rhythms of life.

Managing PMS with Ayurvedic Herbs and Diet

PMS often feels like an unwelcome guest who is unannounced and overstays its welcome. In Ayurveda, PMS is more than just a collection of symptoms; it reflects imbalances in your doshas. Each symptom can be linked to a specific dosha, providing a map to understand what your body is trying to communicate. Pitta imbalances often manifest as irritability and headaches, fueled by excess heat and intensity. You might feel like you're always on edge, ready to snap at the slightest provocation. Meanwhile, Vata imbalances often lead to anxiety and bloating. This leaves you feeling scattered and uneasy, like you're being pulled in many different directions. Understanding these connections can be the first step in finding relief.

Herbal remedies can offer gentle yet effective relief for PMS symptoms. Chamomile and fennel tea, for instance, work wonders as a calming and digestive aid. Sipping a warm cup can soothe your nerves and ease bloating, providing a moment of peace amid the chaos. For those battling inflammation and pain, ginger and turmeric are your allies. Both possess potent anti-inflammatory properties that can mitigate cramps and reduce swelling. Imagine incorporating a simple ginger-turmeric tea into your routine, creating a ritual of care that soothes both body and mind. These herbs don't just mask symptoms; they work with your body to restore balance.

Dietary changes can also play a pivotal role in managing PMS. Vata types might find solace in snacks like nuts and seeds, which are grounding and nourishing. These foods help stabilize the erratic energy that Vata can bring. On the other hand, if Pitta is your dominant dosha, consider incorporating cooling foods like cucumber and watermelon. These choices can counteract the fiery nature of Pitta, offering relief from irritability and heat. By choosing foods that align with your dosha, you create a diet that supports balance and well-being, turning your meals into a powerful tool for health.

Lifestyle practices are equally important in minimizing PMS symptoms. Gentle yoga, with poses designed for relaxation, can offer a sanctuary of calm. Imagine flowing through a series of poses that ease tension and promote relaxation, allowing you to reconnect with your body and mind. Warm baths enhanced with essential oils, such as lavender, can also work wonders. The warm water soothes aching muscles while the aroma of lavender calms your mind and lifts your spirits. These practices invite you to slow down and listen to your body's needs, offering a break from the demands of daily life.

PMS Symptom Tracker

Consider keeping a journal to track your PMS symptoms and the effectiveness of different remedies. Note which symptoms arise, your herbal and dietary choices, and how you feel throughout your cycle. This tracker can become an invaluable tool for understanding your body's rhythms and finding the most effective strategies for relief.

PMS is a complex tapestry woven from the threads of doshic imbalances, lifestyle factors, and emotions. By approaching it with the holistic lens of Ayurveda, you empower yourself to address the root causes rather than just the symptoms. Herbal remedies, mindful dietary choices, and nurturing lifestyle practices offer a path to relief that honors your body's innate wisdom. As you explore these options, you may discover new layers of understanding about yourself, turning PMS from a dreaded monthly visitor into an opportunity for self-care and growth.

Supporting Thyroid Health through Ayurveda

The thyroid, a small butterfly-shaped gland located at the base of your neck, plays a crucial role in regulating hormones that influence your metabolism, energy levels, and overall vitality. From an Ayurvedic perspective, the thyroid's function is closely tied to the balance of doshas—Kapha, Pitta, and Vata. Each dosha brings its own influence on thyroid health. When Kapha becomes imbalanced, it often manifests as hypothyroidism, leading to symptoms like sluggishness, weight gain, and a general feeling of lethargy. This excess of Kapha can create a sense of heaviness, as if the body is moving through thick, viscous fluid. On the other hand, a Vata imbalance might lead to hyperthyroidism, characterized by anxiety, restlessness, and an accelerated heartbeat. Here, the body's energy feels scattered, like leaves swirling in the wind, unable to find a settled state.

Ayurveda offers a gentle yet practical approach to support thyroid health through natural remedies and lifestyle adjustments. Herbs like Guggul and Ashwagandha are particularly beneficial. Guggul, a resin extracted from the Mukul myrrh tree, is recognized for its capacity to support healthy thyroid function and regulate metabolism. It helps clear the body's channels, promoting efficient thyroid activity. Meanwhile, Ashwagandha, a revered adaptogen, helps reduce stress and regulate hormone levels, thereby calming the body and mind. Alongside these herbs, herbal teas like Tulsi and licorice offer additional support. Tulsi, also known as holy basil, acts as a stress reliever and supports the immune system, while licorice helps maintain adrenal health, which is crucial for supporting thyroid function.

Diet is a foundational pillar in Ayurveda, and when it comes to thyroid health, the right foods can make a significant difference. Incorporating iodine-rich foods into your diet is key, as iodine is vital for thyroid hormone production. Add seaweed and fish to your meals, as they are excellent sources of this essential mineral. However, it's also important to be mindful of goitrogenic foods, such as soy and cruciferous vegetables like broccoli and cabbage, which can interfere with thyroid function if consumed in large amounts. Moderation is key, and cooking these vegetables can help reduce their goitrogenic effects, allowing you to enjoy their benefits without compromising your thyroid health.

Lifestyle modifications provide an additional layer of support for thyroid health. Regular exercise, such as walking or swimming, boosts metabolism, helps manage weight, and improves mood. These activities promote circulation and stimulate the body's natural rhythms, aligning with the Ayurvedic principle of movement as medicine. Stress reduction is equally crucial, as chronic stress can wreak havoc on thyroid function. Incorporate meditation and deep breathing exercises into your daily routine to promote relaxation and overall well-being. These practices help calm the mind, reduce anxiety, and create a sense of balance that supports overall well-being. Taking a few minutes each day to focus on your breath can be a transformative practice, offering a respite from the demands of everyday life.

In Ayurveda, routine is viewed as a grounding force, a means to establish stability and predictability in one's life. Creating a daily routine that incorporates time for exercise, mindful eating, and relaxation can make a significant difference. By prioritizing these practices, you create an environment that allows your thyroid to thrive, enabling you to move through your day with energy and ease. As you explore these Ayurvedic approaches to thyroid health, remember that small, consistent changes can lead to significant improvements. Embrace the wisdom of this ancient practice and allow it to guide you towards a state of balance and vitality.

Nurturing Emotional Balance: Ayurvedic Practices for Mood Swings

Emotions can seem like a rollercoaster, especially when hormonal changes are at play. Ayurveda views these emotional fluctuations as reflections of doshic imbalances. When your hormones shift, they can stir the mind, much like wind rippling across a lake, unsettling the surface and the depths. Vata, with its airy and mobile nature, often leads to anxiety and restlessness. Pitta, being fiery, might spark irritability or anger. Meanwhile, Kapha, with its earthy qualities, can result in feelings of heaviness or lethargy. Understanding this connection helps you recognize that mood swings aren't just random; they're signals from your body that it's time to restore balance.

Ayurveda offers various techniques to nurture emotional stability and manage these moods. Breathing exercises, such as alternate nostril breathing, are powerful tools. This practice, known as Nadi Shodhana, calms the mind and balances energy flow, bringing a sense of tranquility. Meditation is another cornerstone of emotional health. Try guided imagery, where you visualize peaceful scenes, or mantra meditation, focusing on repeated phrases that foster calm. These practices anchor you, providing refuge from the storm of emotions. As you engage with these techniques, you may find that the waves of mood swings soften, leaving you more at peace.

Herbs and supplements can also support emotional health, acting as gentle allies in your quest for balance. Brahmi and Shankhpushpi are two such herbs, revered in Ayurveda for their calming properties. Brahmi, often known as the "herb of grace," promotes mental clarity and reduces anxiety. Shankhpushpi, traditionally used to enhance cognitive function, soothes the nervous system, helping you navigate emotional turbulence. In addition to this, consider incorporating omega-3 fatty acids into your diet. These healthy fats, found in fish and flaxseed, support brain health and mood regulation, equipping you with resilience against emotional upheavals.

Self-care is not just a luxury; it's a necessity, especially when emotions run high. Ayurveda emphasizes nurturing oneself through rituals that replenish the spirit. Massages with sesame oil, known as Abhyanga, are deeply soothing. The warmth of the oil, combined with gentle touch, calms the nervous system, releasing tension and grounding your energy. Journaling offers another avenue for self-care. It provides a space to process emotions, transforming your thoughts and feelings into words that can be expressed. This act of reflection can be cathartic, helping you gain insights and clarity. Through these practices, you honor your needs and create a sanctuary of calm amid life's chaos.

As we explore the intricacies of emotional well-being, remember that these practices are not about achieving perfection. They're about creating a supportive environment where you can thrive. By understanding the connection between hormones and emotions, you empower yourself to take proactive steps toward balance. Embrace the tools of Ayurveda, breathing exercises, meditation, herbs, and self-care, as companions on this path. They offer gentle, effective ways to navigate the emotional landscape, helping you cultivate a life filled with peace and resilience.

In this chapter, we've uncovered ways to nurture emotional balance through Ayurveda. We've explored how hormonal changes affect mood and offered strategies to manage them effectively. As you continue, remember that these practices are not just about addressing symptoms but about fostering a deeper connection with yourself. In the next chapter, we'll delve into the heart of Ayurvedic nutrition, exploring how food can be a powerful ally in your quest for holistic health. Together, we'll discover the nourishing power of mindful eating, guiding you toward a balanced and vibrant life.

Chapter 3: Digestive Wellness and Nutrition

In Ayurveda, health begins with what you eat and how well your body digests it. This system of wellness emphasizes selecting foods that cater to your individual needs and promote internal balance. It's not just about the ingredients on your plate, but also about how those foods affect your energy, mood, and overall well-being. By aligning your meals with your body's natural rhythms, you can support better digestion, hormonal health, and long-term vitality.

The core principles of Ayurvedic nutrition revolve around understanding your unique dosha constitution and aligning your diet accordingly. Ayurveda recognizes the power of fresh, seasonal ingredients as the foundation of good health. Consuming foods in their natural season helps you remain in sync with nature's cycles, enhancing digestion and absorption. Imagine biting into a ripe summer peach or savoring a hearty winter root vegetable stew. These choices are about taste and aligning your body's needs with the world around you.

Central to Ayurvedic nutrition is the concept of balancing the six tastes: sweet, sour, salty, bitter, pungent, and astringent. Each taste plays a specific role in health, influencing your doshas and overall well-being. For instance, sweet foods like fruits and grains provide nourishment and grounding, while bitter greens like kale and spinach cleanse and detoxify the body. Sour foods such as citrus fruits aid digestion, while pungent spices like ginger and garlic stimulate appetite and metabolism. Salty foods, used in moderation, help balance electrolytes, while astringent foods like beans and legumes offer a drying and cooling effect.

Spices are highly valued in Ayurveda, serving as both flavor enhancers and medicinal agents. They are crucial in promoting

Agni, the digestive fire that transforms food into energy. Cumin, coriander, and fennel are renowned for their digestive properties. They help alleviate bloating and enhance nutrient absorption, transforming a simple meal into a digestive powerhouse. Black pepper and ginger are known for enhancing metabolic fire. A dash of black pepper can unlock the health benefits of turmeric, while a slice of fresh ginger before a meal can awaken your taste buds and prepare your stomach for digestion.

Eating according to your dosha is a personalized approach that aligns with your body's natural constitution. If you identify with Vata, focus on warm, moist meals that provide comfort and stability. Think of creamy soups, stews, and hearty grains. Pitta types benefit from cooling and hydrating foods. Enjoy salads, fruits, and dairy, which help soothe Pitta's fiery nature. For Kapha, light and dry meals are ideal. Opt for roasted vegetables, legumes, and light grains that invigorate and energize your body.

The timing and routine of meals play a pivotal role in digestion. Ayurveda suggests that your main meal should be consumed at midday when Agni is strongest, much like the sun at its peak. This is when your body can best digest and assimilate nutrients. Conversely, late-night snacking can disrupt digestion and lead to imbalances. It's like asking your body to work overtime when it should be resting and restoring.

Dosha Meal Planning Checklist

Create a checklist to guide your meal planning according to your dosha. List foods and spices that align with your constitution, meal timing preferences, and seasonal adjustments. Use this tool to experiment and discover what combinations make you feel your best.

Incorporating these Ayurvedic dietary guidelines creates a foundation for digestive wellness that nurtures both body and spirit. It's not just about what you eat, but how you honor your body's needs, listen to its signals, and integrate ancient wisdom into your modern life.

Recipes for Reducing Bloating and Indigestion

Bloating after meals is a common issue that can leave you feeling uncomfortable and sluggish. Ayurveda offers practical solutions through simple, natural remedies. One effective option is fennel and mint tea. Fennel seeds are known to support digestion and help reduce gas, while mint has a cooling effect that can ease discomfort. To make the tea, steep one teaspoon of fennel seeds and a few fresh mint leaves in hot water for several minutes. Drink slowly to support digestion and relieve bloating.

Consider a cucumber and dill salad for a refreshing dish that cools and calms the stomach. The crispness of cucumber, known for its hydrating properties, pairs beautifully with the subtle earthiness of dill. This salad not only refreshes but also supports digestion. Toss sliced cucumbers with a sprinkle of dill and a touch of lemon juice. It's a perfect side dish that brings a cooling effect, especially beneficial during warmer months or when your digestive system feels fiery.

Balancing your digestive health isn't just about managing symptoms; it involves nurturing your gut microbiome with prebiotic and probiotic foods. Yogurt with a sprinkle of cumin seeds can be a delightful addition to a meal. Yogurt is rich in probiotics, the beneficial bacteria that help maintain gut health. Meanwhile, cumin is a digestive aid that enhances the benefits of the yogurt. Similarly, incorporating fermented foods like sauerkraut and kefir into your diet can boost your gut flora. These foods are rich in probiotics, which support a healthy digestive system and help reduce the occurrence of bloating and indigestion.

Fiber-rich foods play a vital role in promoting a healthy digestive tract. Lentil soup is a comforting option rich in fiber and protein. Lentils, a staple in Ayurvedic cuisine, provide the bulk necessary to keep your digestive system functioning smoothly. Cook them with spices like turmeric and cumin to create a flavorful and nourishing soup. Whole grains, such as quinoa and brown rice, also support digestion. These grains are rich in fiber and provide essential nutrients that support overall health.

Mindful cooking and eating can transform your dining experience into a practice of self-care. Chewing your food thoroughly is a simple yet powerful technique that aids digestion. It allows your digestive enzymes to break down food more effectively, reducing the likelihood of bloating. As you cook, create a calming environment in your kitchen. Play soothing music, take deep breaths, and focus on the task at hand. Cooking with intention can enhance the nutritional value of your meals, turning them into a form of meditation.

Mindful Eating Reflection Section

Take a moment to reflect on your eating habits. Consider keeping a journal to record your feelings before and after meals. Pay attention to your emotions, the pace at which you eat, and any digestive discomfort you experience. This exercise can help you identify patterns and encourage mindful eating practices.

By incorporating these Ayurvedic recipes and practices into your daily routine, you can support your digestive health and enjoy meals that not only nourish your body but also bring joy and comfort.

Seasonal Eating: Aligning Diet with Ayurvedic Seasons

Ayurveda introduces the concept of Ritucharya, or seasonal routine, a practice that aligns your lifestyle and diet with the changing seasons. Each season carries its energy and characteristics, affecting both the environment and your internal balance. As the seasons transition, so do your doshas, requiring adjustments in your diet to maintain harmony within. It's about listening to the cues of the natural world and responding with care and intention.

In Ayurveda, each season is associated with a specific dosha: Vata, Pitta, or Kapha. The vata season, characterized by cold and dry qualities, calls for warming and grounding foods. Think of hearty stews and root vegetables that provide the warmth your body craves. Pitta season, with its intense heat, requires cooling and hydrating foods. Fresh salads, melons, and cucumbers help soothe the fiery nature of the Pitta—Kapha season, characterized by dampness and heaviness, which benefits from light and stimulating foods. Spicy dishes, light grains, and fresh fruits can invigorate the senses and energize you.

Seasonal transitions have a profound impact on the balance of the doshas. As the weather shifts, your body naturally craves different foods and energy. Embracing these changes helps maintain equilibrium. For instance, as the warmth of summer gives way to the crispness of fall, you may notice a desire for grounding foods that stabilize and nourish. Recognizing and honoring these cravings allows you to remain in sync with your body's needs, promoting overall well-being.

Seasonal cleansing and rejuvenation are vital practices in Ayurveda. They provide an opportunity to reset and renew, clearing out accumulated toxins and revitalizing the body. In spring, a cleanse with herbal teas and detoxifying soups can refresh the system, preparing you for the renewal of life. As fall approaches, nourishing stews and root vegetables offer sustenance, grounding your energy, and fortifying you for the colder months. These practices are not about deprivation but about creating space for growth and transformation.

Aligning your meals with nature's cycles brings a deep sense of connection to the world around you. It highlights the intricate relationship between your body's rhythms and the environment. Eating in harmony with circadian rhythms, such as having meals with daylight cycles, can enhance digestion and energy levels. Imagine enjoying a nourishing breakfast as the sun rises or savoring a light dinner as it sets. These practices support your physical health and nurture your spirit, fostering a sense of unity with the world.

Seasonal Eating Reflection Section

Reflect on your current eating habits and how they align with the seasons. Consider keeping a journal to note any changes in your cravings, energy levels, and overall well-being as the seasons shift. Use this reflection to explore ways to incorporate seasonal eating into your lifestyle, honoring your body's natural rhythms and the world around you.

Mindful Eating: Cultivating a Sattvic Approach to Meals

Imagine a meal that satisfies your hunger and nourishes your soul. This is the promise of the Sattvic approach to eating, a cornerstone of Ayurveda that promotes clarity and inner peace. Sattvic foods are characterized by their light, pure, and fresh nature. They include vibrant fruits, crisp vegetables, whole grains, and nuts. These foods are not just fuel but a source of balance, encouraging a calm and focused mind. By choosing Sattvic foods, you invite harmony into your life, enhancing both your physical and mental well-being.

To fully embrace this approach, consider cultivating mindfulness during meals. Start with a few deep breaths, inhaling slowly and exhaling with intention. This practice centers you, bringing awareness to the present moment. Before you take your first bite, pause to acknowledge the journey your food has taken to reach your plate. This gratitude ritual can be as simple as offering a silent thank you to the earth, the farmers, and the elements that contribute to your meal. Such mindfulness transforms eating from a mundane task into a sacred ritual, deepening your connection to the nourishment you receive.

Your emotional state significantly impacts digestion. Stress, anxiety, and even excitement can affect how your body processes food. Recognizing emotional eating triggers is crucial. Are you reaching for that extra serving because you're hungry or because you're feeling overwhelmed? Creating a positive mealtime environment helps. Set an intention for your meal, whether it's to nourish yourself, enjoy the experience, or express gratitude. A calming atmosphere invites relaxation, allowing your digestive system to function optimally. When you eat with awareness, you honor your body's signals, paving the way for better health.

Some Sattvic meals exemplify this philosophy beautifully. Vegetable khichdi, for instance, is a simple and nourishing dish that embodies balance. It's made from mung beans and rice, gently spiced with turmeric and cumin. This one-pot meal is easy to digest, making it an ideal choice for those seeking a balanced diet. For a lighter option, consider a fresh fruit salad. For a refreshing dish, combine seasonal fruits like apples, grapes, and pomegranate seeds. A drizzle of honey or a sprinkle of cinnamon adds a touch of sweetness, enhancing the natural flavors of the dish.

Gratitude Practice for Meals

Take a moment before each meal to practice gratitude. Reflect on the journey of your food, from seed to plate. Consider writing down your thoughts in a journal, noting how this practice influences your dining experience and emotional well-being.

Each meal offers an opportunity to practice mindfulness and embrace the Sattvic approach. By choosing foods that promote clarity and peace, you nourish not only your body but also your mind and spirit.

Kitchari Cleanses: A Gentle Detox for Women

Kitchari, pronounced "kich-uh-ree," is often considered the cornerstone of Ayurvedic cleansing. Imagine a dish that is satisfying, deeply nourishing, and detoxifying—a gentle reset for your digestive system. This humble dish blends mung beans and basmati rice, cooked together to create a soft, porridge-like consistency. The magic of Kitchari lies in its simplicity and balance. It provides a perfect combination of protein, carbohydrates, and healthy fats, making it a nutrient-dense and easily digestible food. This is why Kitchari is the go-to food for those seeking a gentle detox that doesn't leave you feeling deprived.

Preparing Kitchari is a ritual that invites you to slow down and connect with the healing properties of your food.

- Begin by rinsing ½ cup of split yellow mung beans and ½ cup of basmati rice under cold running water.
- In a pot, heat a tablespoon of ghee and add a teaspoon of each of the cumin seeds, coriander seeds, and turmeric.
- Let the spices sizzle and fill the air with their warm, earthy aroma.
- Add the rinsed mung beans, rice, and four cups of water.
- Bring it to a boil, then reduce the heat to a simmer, cover the pot, and allow it to cook until the mixture is soft and creamy.
- For Vata doshas, add extra ginger and black pepper to warm and ground the dish.
- Pitta doshas might prefer a cooling garnish of cilantro and a squeeze of lime.
- Kapha doshas can spice things up with a pinch of cayenne or a dash of mustard seeds.

The benefits of a Kitchari cleanse extend beyond its nutritional profile. Its gentle nature makes it ideal for resetting your digestive system, particularly after periods of indulgence or stress. Kitchari is incredibly easy to digest, allowing your body to focus on eliminating toxins rather than breaking down complex foods. The mung beans, in particular, possess detoxifying properties that support liver function and aid in cleansing the digestive tract. Imagine your body as a garden, one that needs occasional weeding and nurturing to flourish. A Kitchari cleanse offers this, providing a nurturing space for your digestive health to bloom.

Incorporating Kitchari into your cleansing routine can be a rewarding practice. Aim for three to seven days of cleansing, depending on your body's needs. During this time, support your cleanse with herbal teas like ginger or peppermint, which aid digestion and soothe the stomach. Gentle yoga practices can enhance detox, encouraging your body to release tension and toxins. As you embark on your cleanse, listen to your body's signals. If you feel tired, rest. If you're thirsty, hydrate with warm water or herbal tea. This is your time to tune in and honor your body's innate wisdom.

Consider these tips for maximizing the effectiveness of your Kitchari cleanse: First, focus on mindfulness during meals. Before each bite, take a moment to breathe deeply and express gratitude for your food. This practice enhances digestion and fosters a sense of peace and contentment. Second, create a supportive environment. Surround yourself with calming music, soft lighting, and comfortable seating. These elements transform your meal into a nourishing ritual, both for your body and your spirit. Finally, allow yourself the grace to adapt the cleanse to your unique needs. If you're feeling cold, add warming spices. If you're craving variety, experiment with different vegetables or herbs to add a unique twist to your dishes. Kitchari is a flexible dish that can be tailored to your dosha and personal preferences, making it a truly personalized cleanse.

As you adopt the practice of Kitchari cleansing, you may experience a renewed sense of vitality and balance within. This simple, nourishing dish offers a gateway to a deeper connection with your body and its needs, encouraging you to cultivate a lifestyle of mindful nourishment.

Incorporating Superfoods: Turmeric, Ashwagandha, and More

Ayurveda highlights certain ingredients, such as turmeric, ashwagandha, and triphala, for their powerful health benefits. These natural substances are valued for their ability to support immunity, reduce inflammation, improve digestion, and promote overall balance in the body.

Let's explore how these ancient ingredients can be seamlessly woven into your daily life. Turmeric, with its golden hue, is celebrated for its anti-inflammatory and antioxidant properties. It's like a natural shield, protecting your body from the wear and tear of daily life while enhancing your immune response. A warm cup of turmeric golden milk, made by simmering turmeric with milk and spices like cinnamon and black pepper, is comforting and nourishing, especially on those chilly evenings when you need a little extra warmth.

Ashwagandha, often called the "king of Ayurveda," is an adaptogen, a class of herbs that helps the body adapt to stress and maintain balance. Blending it into your morning smoothie, along with bananas and almond milk, can energize your day while keeping you calm and focused.

Triphala, a combination of three fruits (amla, bibhitaki, and haritaki), is renowned for its digestive health and detoxification benefits. Picture it as a gentle cleanser sweeping through your digestive system and keeping it clean and efficient. A teaspoon mixed with warm water before bed can aid in regular bowel movements, ensuring you wake up feeling refreshed and light.

When incorporating these superfoods into your diet, sourcing quality products is crucial. Organic and sustainably sourced options ensure that the ingredients retain their potency and purity, free from harmful chemicals and additives. This guarantees that you're supporting your health and honoring the environment. When purchasing, look for reputable brands with transparent sourcing practices. This way, you can trust that what's on the label truly benefits your health.

The beauty of superfoods lies in their synergy with Ayurvedic practices. They don't just stand alone; they complement and enhance your holistic health routines. Start your day with a morning ritual with a turmeric-infused tea, setting a tone of warmth and healing. As evening falls, unwind with an ashwagandha tea, letting its calming properties ease you into relaxation. These small practices integrate seamlessly into your day, harmonizing the body, mind, and spirit.

Incorporating superfoods into your lifestyle is more than just a health fad; it's about reconnecting with ancient wisdom that has stood the test of time. These ingredients offer more than just nutritional benefits; they're a reminder of the simplicity and power of nature.

As we close this chapter on digestive wellness, remember that each choice you make in your diet and lifestyle has the power to nurture and transform. These principles of Ayurveda offer guidance not just for your body but for your entire being. In the next chapter, we'll explore the connection between movement and wellness, delving into yoga and exercise as tools for enhancing your health. Let's continue to embrace the wisdom of Ayurveda, weaving these practices into a life of balance, vitality, and joy.

Chapter 4: Life Stage Transitions and Ayurveda

Fertility and Ayurveda: Enhancing Reproductive Health

In Ayurveda, fertility is supported by maintaining balance throughout the body and mind. Reproductive health improves when key areas such as digestion, sleep, and stress are addressed with consistency and care. Ayurveda encourages gradual lifestyle changes—such as reducing stress and maintaining a regular sleep routine—as part of a holistic approach to fertility. For example, incorporating calming habits like drinking a warm herbal tea before bed can help support hormonal balance and overall well-being.

Diet plays a pivotal role in promoting fertility. Ayurveda encourages you to savor foods that nourish your body and support reproductive health. Picture a handful of almonds and pumpkin seeds, rich in essential nutrients, becoming a staple in your daily routine. These foods, rich in healthy fats and vitamins, support your body's fertility potential. At the same time, steering clear of processed foods and excessive caffeine can make a world of difference. Think of it as clearing weeds from a garden, allowing your body to flourish without interference.

Ayurvedic herbs and treatments offer natural remedies to enhance fertility. Ashwagandha, known for its adaptogenic properties, helps support hormonal balance by reducing stress and anxiety. Envision blending it into a warm beverage, its earthy flavor grounding your spirit. Shatavari, often called the "queen of herbs," nurtures reproductive health. Its soothing properties balance hormones and support the reproductive organs. Fertility massages, targeting the abdominal area, stimulate the reproductive organs, encouraging circulation and nourishment.

Emotional well-being is intricately connected to fertility, emphasizing the importance of maintaining emotional balance. Techniques like art therapy or guided imagery offer creative outlets for emotional release. Imagine expressing your hopes and dreams through vibrant strokes of color on a canvas, translating feelings into art. Stress management practices, such as yoga and meditation, become anchors of calm in your life. Visualize yourself in a quiet space, focusing on your breath, allowing stress to dissipate with each exhale. Though simple, these practices can transform your emotional landscape, supporting fertility from the inside out.

Emotional Well-Being Reflection Section

Consider setting aside time each week to reflect on your emotional well-being. Use this space to explore your feelings, document changes, and celebrate moments of growth. This practice can deepen your connection to yourself and provide clarity as you navigate your fertility journey.

Pregnancy

Pregnancy is a significant phase in a woman's life, characterized by physical, emotional, and hormonal changes. In Ayurveda, this time is approached with care and intention, focusing on supporting both the mother and the developing baby. The goal is to maintain balance and promote well-being through proper nutrition, rest, and emotional support. Ayurveda offers a holistic approach that addresses the needs of the body, mind, and spirit during pregnancy, helping to create a healthy environment for both mother and child.

Ayurveda recommends a Sattvic diet during pregnancy, which involves focusing on fresh, organic produce that nourishes both the mother and the baby. Imagine savoring ripe fruits, vibrant vegetables, and wholesome grains, all chosen for their purity and vitality. These foods provide the essential nutrients your body craves, supporting the growth and development of your baby. It's about filling your plate with goodness that uplifts your spirit and nourishes your body, creating a foundation of health and wellness for both of you.

Pregnancy yoga provides an additional layer of support, introducing gentle asanas that promote relaxation and ease. These movements are not about exertion but about finding comfort in your changing body. Picture yourself moving through poses that open your hips, ease tension in your back, and connect you with your breath. This practice becomes a sacred time for you and your baby, allowing you to tune into your body's needs and embrace the changes with grace. It's a reminder that pregnancy is not just a physical journey, but a spiritual one as well.

Dietary recommendations in Ayurveda evolve with each trimester, recognizing your body's unique needs as your pregnancy progresses. In the first trimester, light, warm foods can ease the nausea that often accompanies early pregnancy. Imagine sipping on nourishing broths or enjoying simple rice dishes that calm your stomach and provide comfort. Nutrient-dense meals become crucial as you enter the second trimester, supporting your baby's growth. Think of colorful salads sprinkled with seeds, or hearty stews filled with legumes and greens, all crafted to nourish and sustain.

In the third trimester, easy-to-digest foods offer comfort and support as your body prepares for birth. Warm porridge, gentle soups, and steamed vegetables provide sustenance without overwhelming your digestion. It's about honoring your body's wisdom, choosing foods that soothe and sustain as you approach the final stages of pregnancy.

Ayurveda also offers remedies for common pregnancy discomforts, helping you easily navigate the challenges. Ginger tea becomes a trusted ally, soothing nausea with its warming properties. For swelling and fatigue, warm sesame oil massages provide relief, melting away tension and inviting relaxation. These practices become a sanctuary, offering moments of peace and rejuvenation.

Emotional well-being is equally important during pregnancy, and Ayurveda provides tools to nurture your mental health. Meditation and breathing exercises become daily rituals, offering a refuge from stress and anxiety. Picture yourself sitting in stillness, focusing on your breath, allowing worries to drift away. Positive affirmations and visualization techniques further support emotional health, encouraging a mindset of strength and positivity. By envisioning a healthy, joyful pregnancy, you create space for these qualities to manifest in your life.

Pregnancy Reflection Section

Consider keeping a pregnancy journal, a space to record your thoughts, feelings, and experiences. Reflect on the changes in your body, the emotions that arise, and your dreams for your child. This practice fosters a deeper connection with yourself and your baby and creates a cherished keepsake for years to come.

Through Ayurveda, pregnancy becomes a time of nurturing and growth, where each choice you make supports your and your baby's health and well-being.

Postpartum Care: Rejuvenation and Recovery

In the whirlwind of new motherhood, the postpartum phase is a sacred time, one that Ayurveda cherishes deeply. It's a period of immense change, where rest and rejuvenation are encouraged and essential. Your body has just accomplished an incredible feat, and now it's time to focus on healing and restoring balance. Ayurveda places great importance on this stage, emphasizing practices that nourish and soothe both body and soul. Restorative practices like abhyanga, an ancient oil massage, become a daily ritual. Imagine warm oil enveloping your skin, its soothing touch melting away fatigue and tension, inviting relaxation and healing.

Nourishment is equally vital during postpartum recovery. Your body, now tasked with healing and providing for your newborn, craves grounding and rejuvenating sustenance. Warm, cooked meals like kichari and dal become staples, and their gentle flavors and nourishing ingredients provide comfort and strength. These meals are food and medicine, supporting your body's natural processes and enhancing your energy. Galactagogue herbs like fenugreek and fennel are also introduced, and they are known for their ability to promote lactation and support postpartum recovery. Get your pantry stocked with these supportive herbs, ready to be brewed into soothing teas or added to meals, offering gentle, healing support.

Self-care during this time is not just a luxury; it's a necessity. Carving out moments for yourself can feel challenging, yet it's crucial for your well-being. Gentle yoga and stretching become allies in your recovery, helping you reconnect with your body and restore physical strength. Transform a quiet corner of your home into a nurturing space where you can stretch and breathe, releasing the day's stresses. Herbal baths provide another layer of self-care, their fragrant waters inviting relaxation and rejuvenation. Envision yourself soaking in a warm bath infused with calming herbs, allowing their soothing properties to envelop your senses and promote relaxation and healing.

Emotionally, the postpartum period can be a rollercoaster, with mood swings and emotional shifts often taking center stage. Ayurveda recognizes this and offers practices to support mental health during this time. Engaging with support networks, such as other mothers, provides invaluable connection and understanding. Imagine sharing stories, laughter, and tears with those who are walking similar paths, finding comfort and camaraderie in shared experiences. Journaling becomes a powerful tool for emotional processing, offering a safe space to explore your feelings. As your pen glides across the page, you might find clarity and insight, transforming complex emotions into words that make sense of the chaos.

In these early days of motherhood, balancing caring for your newborn and nurturing yourself is delicate. Yet, it's essential to remember that by caring for yourself, you are, in turn, caring for your baby. Through Ayurveda's lens, the postpartum period is a time of renewal and healing, where rest, nourishment, and self-care form the foundation of recovery. Embrace these practices not just as tasks to be checked off, but as acts of love and devotion to yourself and your new role as a mother.

Navigating Menopause Naturally with Ayurvedic Support

As you enter menopause, Ayurveda views menopause as a powerful opportunity for transformation and self-discovery. It's a natural transition, one that invites you to embrace the changes with curiosity and openness. Menopause, often aligned with the Vata stage of life, encourages you to welcome the shifts gracefully. Vata's airy and mobile qualities can bring about feelings of dryness and anxiety. However, you can navigate this stage with poise by aligning with Ayurvedic principles.

To ease menopause symptoms like hot flashes and mood swings, Ayurveda suggests embracing cooling herbs such as Shatavari and Brahmi. These herbs work gently to soothe the fiery discomfort that can arise. Imagine sipping a calming tea infused with Brahmi and feeling its cooling essence calm your mind and body. Lifestyle practices such as cooling pranayama help manage internal heat, while meditation offers a sanctuary of peace amidst the changes. Picture yourself in a quiet space, breathing deeply, as you let go of tension and welcome tranquility into your being.

Dietary adjustments can also significantly contribute to menopausal health. Vata-pacifying foods, like root vegetables and ghee, provide grounding and nourishment. Imagine savoring a warm bowl of roasted sweet potatoes, their earthy sweetness comforting your senses. Calcium-rich foods like sesame seeds and leafy greens bolster bone health, ensuring strength as you move through this stage. Think of a vibrant salad topped with toasted sesame seeds, each bite reinforcing your bones and vitality.

Emotional resilience and self-exploration become key components of this transition. Reflective journaling allows you to explore new life stages and embrace the wisdom gained through experience. Envision your thoughts flowing onto the pages, creating insights and understanding. Community engagement, such as joining support groups, offers connection and shared experiences. Picture a circle of women, each sharing their stories, finding strength in their collective wisdom. These practices foster a sense of belonging and acceptance, reminding you that you are not alone on this path.

Menopause Reflection Section

Consider setting aside time each week to reflect on your experiences during menopause. Use this space to explore your emotions, document changes, and celebrate moments of growth. This practice can deepen your connection to yourself and provide clarity as you navigate this transformative phase.

Menopause marks a time of renewal, an invitation to rediscover yourself and embrace the richness of life. With Ayurveda's gentle guidance, you can move through this period with confidence and grace, honoring the natural rhythm of your body and spirit.

Supporting Bone Health in Aging Women

As you age, maintaining bone health becomes increasingly vital. From an Ayurvedic perspective, bone health isn't just about physical structure; it's about a balanced life, where mind, body, and spirit work together to support your well-being. Preventive care takes center stage, and it begins with early intervention. Establishing healthy habits early on can serve as a strong foundation for your later years. Ayurveda places great value on nurturing these habits, focusing on a holistic approach that includes diet, exercise, and lifestyle to keep bones strong and resilient.

Diet plays a crucial role in supporting bone health. Calcium-rich foods like sesame seeds and almonds are more than just delicious; they're powerful allies in maintaining bone density. Enjoy the nutty crunch of sesame seeds sprinkled over a vibrant salad or the creamy taste of almond butter spread on whole-grain bread. These simple additions to your diet can make a significant impact. For those who prefer dairy alternatives, almond milk and tofu offer excellent sources of calcium. Their versatility allows them to be seamlessly integrated into your meals, providing nourishment and support to your bones.

Ayurvedic treatments and exercises further enhance bone strength. Weight-bearing activities, such as walking and yoga, are not just about staying active; they also stimulate bone growth and maintain bone density. Imagine a morning walk, the sun warming your skin, as you stride with purpose, each step strengthening your bones. Yoga, with its gentle stretches and poses, provides an additional layer of support, promoting flexibility and balance. In addition to exercise, herbal supplements like Cissus quadrangularis and turmeric are recommended for their bone-supporting properties.

Lifestyle modifications are equally necessary in maintaining bone health. Sun exposure is essential for vitamin D synthesis, which aids in calcium absorption. A daily morning walk, even if brief, can provide your body with the sunlight it needs. Feel the morning rays on your face as you stroll, knowing you're nourishing your bones naturally. Stress, often an overlooked factor, can also impact bone health. Incorporating mindfulness and meditation into your routine can help reduce stress, creating a peaceful environment for your body to thrive. Picture yourself in a quiet room, eyes closed, taking deep breaths as you let go of stress, inviting calm and balance into your life.

Bone Health Checklist

Consider creating a checklist to track your bone health practices. Include daily activities such as sun exposure, healthy dietary choices, and stress-reducing exercises. This checklist can serve as a gentle reminder of the small steps you take each day to support your bones.

As you embrace these practices, remember that maintaining bone health is a lifelong commitment. With Ayurveda's holistic approach, you create a foundation that supports not just your bones but your entire being. For more in-depth information and advice, check out my book, Thrive with Osteoporosis.

Embracing the Wisdom Years: Ayurveda for Senior Women

Ayurveda views this phase not as a decline but as an opportunity to celebrate accumulated wisdom and life experiences. These years are about embracing the stories etched in your heart, recognizing the lessons learned, and sharing those with others. They offer a unique perspective, one where the focus shifts from doing to being, from accumulating to appreciating. Embracing wisdom means cherishing the journey that has brought you here and recognizing the unique beauty in each wrinkle and each gray hair.

To support vitality in these years, Ayurveda recommends an anti-inflammatory diet rich in foods like turmeric and ginger. These spices not only add flavor but also help combat inflammation, promoting overall well-being. Imagine a warm cup of ginger tea, each sip soothing and invigorating, or a sprinkle of turmeric in your meals, adding a golden hue and a dose of health. Hydration and fiber-rich foods, such as fresh fruits and vegetables, are essential for maintaining energy and overall health. Picture a colorful plate filled with crisp apples, juicy berries, and crunchy greens, nourishing your body and enlivening your spirit.

Mental and emotional health take on new significance in the wisdom years, offering opportunities for growth and connection. Engaging in activities stimulating the mind, such as puzzles or learning new skills, keeps cognitive faculties sharp. Imagine the satisfaction of completing a challenging puzzle or mastering a new hobby, each moment a testament to your lifelong ability to learn. Emotional well-being thrives when social ties are maintained and connections are nurtured. Picture lively conversations with friends, sharing laughter and stories, each interaction a reminder of the joys of companionship and community.

Spiritual practices can provide support and clarity during times of stress or transition. Regular meditation and mindfulness help calm the mind, improve focus, and promote emotional balance. Setting aside a few minutes each day for quiet reflection can have a meaningful impact on your overall well-being. Joining a spiritual or meditation group may also be helpful, offering a sense of connection and shared understanding through group discussions or guided sessions.

As this chapter draws to a close, remember the wisdom years are not just a time of reflection but a celebration of life's richness. They invite you to embrace the past, cherish the present, and look forward to the future with open arms. With Ayurveda as your guide, these years can be filled with vitality, connection, and peace. As we transition to the next chapter, we will explore integrating these practices into a holistic lifestyle, weaving them into the fabric of daily life for a balanced and fulfilling existence.

Chapter 5: Spiritual and Cultural Integration

Meditation is a core part of Ayurvedic self-care, offering a way to calm the mind and restore balance. It is seen not just as a technique, but as a tool for self-awareness and emotional clarity. By taking a few quiet moments each day to focus on your breath and let go of distractions, you can reduce stress, improve focus, and support overall mental and physical well-being. In Ayurveda, regular meditation helps create a stable, centered state of mind, which is essential for maintaining health and balance.

Meditation holds a place of immense importance in Ayurveda, serving as a cornerstone for mental clarity and emotional balance. Whether you're navigating the stresses of everyday life or seeking a deeper connection with your inner self, meditation provides a refuge. There are various forms of meditation to explore, each offering unique ways to quiet the mind. Vipassana, often referred to as insight meditation, encourages you to observe your thoughts without judgment, thereby fostering a deeper understanding of your mind's workings. Conversely, guided imagery takes you on a mental journey, using vivid visuals to cultivate relaxation and focus. The benefits of meditation extend beyond stress reduction; it enhances concentration and emotional resilience, equipping you with tools to face life's challenges with grace and poise.

Mantras also play a vital role in Ayurvedic healing, serving as powerful tools for transformation. These sacred sounds or phrases resonate with your energy, influencing your mental state and emotional well-being. Consider the mantra "Om," a primordial sound that embodies the essence of the universe. Chanting creates a calming vibration, aligning you with the cosmic rhythm. Another popular mantra, "So Hum," translates to

"I am that," reminding you of your connection to the universe and your intrinsic wholeness. Reciting mantras can be a soothing practice, helping to calm the mind and promote relaxation, much like a lullaby for the soul.

Incorporating meditation and mantras into your daily routine doesn't have to be daunting. Start each day with a short meditation session, setting intentions that align with your goals and values. As you breathe deeply, visualize your aspirations unfolding, planting seeds of positivity for the day ahead. As you prepare for rest, turn to mantra practice in the evening. Allow the rhythmic repetition to quiet your mind, easing the day's tensions and inviting peaceful slumber. These practices fit seamlessly into your routine, nurturing your spirit without overwhelming your schedule.

Creating a conducive environment for meditation enhances the experience, allowing you to immerse yourself in the practice entirely. Find a quiet space free from distractions, where you can retreat from the world and focus inward. Comfortable seating is essential; consider using cushions or blankets to support your body and encourage relaxation. A small altar with meaningful objects, such as crystals or a candle, can further enrich your meditation space, creating an atmosphere of tranquility and reverence.

Personal Meditation Mantra

Take a moment to choose a personal mantra that resonates with you. Reflect on its meaning and how it aligns with your intentions. Write down your mantra and place it in your meditation space as a reminder of your commitment to inner peace. Consider how this practice might transform your daily life, offering a sanctuary of calm amid the chaos.

These practices invite you to explore the depths of your consciousness, fostering a deeper connection with your inner self and the world around you. Embrace the transformative power of meditation and mantras, allowing them to guide you toward a life of balance and serenity.

Understanding Chakras: Energy Centers and Women's Health

In the heart of Ayurvedic philosophy lies the concept of chakras, these invisible yet powerful energy centers that line our spine. Imagine them as spinning wheels of energy, each playing a critical role in our physical and emotional well-being. There are seven major chakras: the root, sacral, solar plexus, heart, throat, third eye, and crown. Each chakra corresponds to specific aspects of our lives, influencing everything from our sense of security to our capacity for love and connection. When these chakras are aligned and balanced, they contribute to a harmonious flow of energy throughout your body, promoting health and vitality. But when blocked or imbalanced, they can manifest as physical ailments or emotional turmoil, suggesting the need for realignment.

The sacral chakra, located in the lower abdomen, is particularly significant for women. It governs reproductive health and creativity, acting as the source of your emotional and sexual energy. Balancing supports a vibrant and expressive life, enhancing your ability to embrace pleasure and joy. However, an imbalance might present as issues with fertility, hormonal imbalances, or creative blocks. Similarly, the heart chakra, nestled at the center of your chest, is the seat of love and emotional openness. A balanced heart chakra fosters compassion and connection, whereas an imbalance may lead to feelings of isolation or a lack of empathy. Chakras are not just mystical concepts but are integral to understanding the interplay between your physical and emotional states.

Balancing and aligning your chakras can be a transformative practice, opening pathways to improved health and well-being. Chakra meditation is a focused way to bring awareness and energy to each center, allowing you to tune into their unique frequencies. This practice often involves visualizing each chakra as a spinning wheel of light, using colors associated with each one to enhance the experience. For instance, envisioning a vibrant orange glow at your sacral chakra can help energize and balance this center, promoting creativity and intimacy. Color therapy further supports chakra health by integrating these hues into your environment, whether through clothing, décor, or even the foods you consume.

Recognizing chakra imbalances involves tuning into your body's signals and emotional cues. You may notice fatigue, emotional instability, or specific physical symptoms that correspond to certain chakras. For example, frequent feelings of insecurity or anxiety might suggest an issue with the root chakra, which governs your sense of safety and grounding. To correct these imbalances, incorporate practices such as yoga poses and affirmations into your daily routine. Poses like Warrior II can ground and stabilize the root chakra, while heart-opening poses like Camel Pose can enhance energy flow through the heart chakra. Affirmations, repeated with intention, reinforce positive energy and healing. A simple affirmation for the heart chakra might be, "I am open to giving and receiving love."

Chakra Health Checklist

Consider creating a checklist to track your chakra health. List each chakra, its associated color, and a few key imbalance symptoms. Note any beneficial practices, such as specific yoga poses or meditations. This tool can be a personal guide, helping you maintain balance and awareness in your energetic body. Keep it in a place where you can easily refer to it, such as your journal or meditation space.

Chakras offer a lens through which you can explore holistic health, connecting the physical and emotional aspects of your being. You can navigate your wellness journey with greater insight and clarity through awareness and attunement, embracing a life of balance and harmony. If you're interested in exploring Chakras in more detail, check out my book, Chakra Healing and the Vagus Nerve.

Exploring Pranayama: Yogic Breathing for Stress Relief

Imagine sitting comfortably, your eyes gently closed, focusing entirely on the rhythm of your breath. This is the essence of Pranayama, an ancient practice in Ayurveda centered on breath regulation to connect the body and mind. "Prana" refers to life energy, while "Yama" means control. Together, they form a vital technique for managing stress and enhancing vitality. In the hustle and bustle of daily life, stress often feels like an unwelcome companion. Pranayama offers a sanctuary, a way to quiet the mind and invigorate the body. With each breath, you draw in energy and release tension, creating a flow of life force that revitalizes you from within.

Among the various techniques, Anulom Vilom, or alternate nostril breathing, stands out for its simplicity and effectiveness. Start by sitting comfortably with your spine straight. Use your right thumb to close your right nostril, and inhale deeply through your left nostril. Close the left nostril with your ring finger, release the right, and exhale gently. Inhale through the right, switch again, and exhale through the left. This rhythmic alternation harmonizes the two hemispheres of your brain, promoting mental clarity and emotional equilibrium. Bhramari, also known as humming bee breath, offers another path to relaxation. Sit comfortably, close your eyes, and cover your ears with your thumbs. Inhale deeply, then exhale slowly while gently humming, reminiscent of a bee. This vibration soothes the mind, quieting the chatter and inviting a sense of calm.

The benefits of Pranayama extend far beyond stress relief. Mentally, it sharpens concentration, allowing you to approach tasks with renewed focus. It's as if a fog lifts, revealing a world of possibilities with remarkable clarity. Physically, regular practice enhances lung capacity and improves respiratory function. Your breaths become deeper and more efficient, fueling your body with the oxygen it craves. This increased lung capacity supports endurance, whether you're hiking up a mountain or simply climbing the stairs. The combination of mental and physical benefits creates a holistic sense of well-being, enabling you to navigate life's challenges with confidence.

Incorporating Pranayama into your routine is a gift to yourself. Morning is an opportune time, as the world awakens around you. Begin with a few rounds of Anulom Vilom to set a calm and balanced tone for the day. As evening falls, wind down with Bhramari, allowing the soothing vibrations to wash away the day's stresses. Consistency is key; even a few minutes daily can create profound changes. As you become more attuned to your breath, you'll find a deeper connection to yourself, a quiet strength that anchors you amid life's chaos.

Creating a space for Pranayama enhances the experience. Choose a quiet corner where you can sit undisturbed. Surround yourself with comfort, perhaps a soft cushion or a blanket to keep you warm. Consider lighting a candle or placing a plant nearby to add a touch of nature's serenity. These simple elements transform your practice into a ritual, a sacred moment of self-care. As you settle in, let go of expectations and be present with your breath. Allow the world to fall away, if only for a moment, as you explore the depths of your own inner landscape.

Pranayama Practice Reflection

Consider keeping a journal to reflect on your Pranayama practice. Note any shifts in your mood, energy levels, or overall well-being. This reflection can help you track your progress and deepen your connection to the practice.

Cultivating Mindfulness: Integrating Ayurveda into Daily Life

Mindfulness is like a gentle whisper, reminding you to be present in each moment. In the world of Ayurveda, mindfulness isn't just a practice; it's a way of living that invites you to be fully engaged in life. Imagine savoring each bite during a meal, truly tasting the flavors and textures. This is mindful eating, a practice that transforms nourishment into an act of self-care. By slowing down and being present, you allow your body to digest food and experiences, creating a more profound sense of satisfaction and well-being. It's about being aware of your surroundings, actions, and thoughts, turning everyday activities into moments of meditation.

The benefits of mindfulness extend to every aspect of your life, enhancing your mental, emotional, and physical well-being. On a mental level, mindfulness helps regulate emotions, offering tools to manage stress and anxiety effectively. It's like having a personal compass that guides you through turbulent waters, allowing you to respond rather than react. Emotionally, mindfulness fosters resilience, helping you navigate life's challenges with a steady heart. Physically, the practice improves digestion, as being present during meals aids digestion. It also enhances sleep quality, as a calm mind is more likely to drift into restful slumber. When you live mindfully, you experience life more fully, finding joy in simplicity and presence in action.

Integrating mindfulness into your daily routine doesn't require an overhaul; it's about small, intentional shifts. Consider starting with mindful walking. As you stroll, focus on the sensations under your feet, the rhythm of your breath, and the world around you. This simple act grounds you, turning an ordinary walk into a moving meditation. Mindful communication is another area to explore. Practice active listening by being fully present when others speak, absorbing their words without distraction. In your work life, embrace mindfulness by focusing on one task at a time, setting aside distractions like phones and social media. This enhances productivity and reduces stress, as your mind is not constantly pulled in multiple directions.

Creating a mindful lifestyle involves weaving these practices into various aspects of your life. Start your day with a few moments of quiet reflection, setting an intention for how you wish to engage with the world. This intention becomes a guiding light, reminding you to return to the present throughout the day. As you move through your routine, pause periodically to check in with yourself. Are you rushing through tasks, or can you savor the moment? These check-ins help recalibrate your focus, ensuring you stay aligned with your goals and intentions. Mindfulness isn't about perfection; it's about being aware and making choices. It's about being gentle with yourself when you stray and celebrating when you return.

Creating a mindful lifestyle is an invitation to slow down and savor life. It's about infusing your actions with presence, whether cooking a meal, conversing, or simply taking a breath. Integrating mindfulness into your daily life creates a foundation of peace and presence, supporting your journey toward holistic health and well-being. As you embrace mindfulness, you'll find that the world becomes richer, your experiences deeper, and your connection to yourself and others more profound. Each moment becomes an opportunity to be present, to engage fully, and to live with intention.

Cultural Sensitivity: Respectful Practice of Ayurveda

When you first encounter Ayurveda, it's like stepping into a world rich with history and tradition. This ancient practice, rooted in the Indian subcontinent, offers a holistic approach to health and wellness. Yet, as you explore its teachings, cultural sensitivity becomes crucial. Understanding the origins of Ayurveda is not just about knowledge; it's about honoring and respecting the wisdom passed down through generations. This involves recognizing the historical context and appreciating the cultural nuances that shape its practice. Engaging with Ayurveda respectfully means acknowledging its roots and ensuring our practices reflect an authentic understanding.

Integrating Ayurveda into modern life requires more than enthusiasm; it demands a thoughtful approach to cultural appreciation and understanding. One of the first steps is learning from authentic sources. Seek guidance from experienced Ayurvedic practitioners who can provide insights into traditional practices. Their wisdom can help you navigate the rich tapestry of Ayurvedic knowledge with respect and accuracy. It's also important to use respectful language, ensuring that the terminology you adopt is precise and honors the tradition. Avoid oversimplifying or misrepresenting concepts for the sake of convenience. Instead, celebrate the complexity and depth that make Ayurveda unique.

The benefits are profound when you engage with Ayurveda in a culturally sensitive manner. Your practice deepens, enriched by a genuine understanding of Ayurvedic principles. This respect for tradition enhances your personal journey, fostering a connection that transcends superficial engagement. By embracing cultural appreciation, you also contribute to a respectful dialogue within the community. This dialogue encourages mutual understanding and learning, allowing Ayurveda to be a bridge between cultures rather than a source of division. Respectful practice enriches your experience and strengthens the community around you, creating a space where diverse voices are valued and celebrated.

To further your understanding of Ayurvedic culture, consider immersing yourself in resources that offer authentic insights and perspectives. Classic texts, such as the "Charaka Samhita" and the "Ashtanga Hridaya," provide foundational knowledge and context. These texts, written centuries ago, remain relevant, offering timeless wisdom on health and wellness. Additionally, community involvement can be a valuable asset. Attend workshops and seminars to learn from seasoned practitioners and enthusiasts alike. These gatherings provide an opportunity to deepen your knowledge and connect with others who share your passion for Ayurveda. They also provide a platform for exchanging ideas and experiences, fostering a sense of community and belonging.

For those eager to explore further, abundant opportunities exist to expand your understanding of Ayurveda. Look into courses that delve into its philosophy, practices, and applications. These courses often provide a structured approach to learning, guiding you step-by-step through the complexities of Ayurvedic thought. Online forums and discussion groups can also be a treasure trove of information and support. Engaging with these communities allows you to share experiences, ask questions, and learn from others who are on a similar path. This collective wisdom, drawn from diverse backgrounds and perspectives, enriches your journey and broadens your horizons.

Incorporating Ayurveda into your life with cultural sensitivity is not a static achievement but an ongoing practice. It requires openness, curiosity, and a willingness to learn and grow. By approaching Ayurveda with respect and humility, you honor its legacy and ensure its teachings remain vibrant and relevant in today's world. This respectful engagement benefits you and contributes to the preservation and appreciation of an ancient tradition that has much to offer in our quest for holistic health and well-being.

Personal Empowerment through Ayurvedic Rituals

Ayurvedic rituals are more than just routine; they are pathways to personal empowerment. Engaging in these rituals fosters a deep sense of self-awareness and personal growth, inviting you to connect meaningfully with your inner self. Imagine starting your day purposefully, tuning into your body's needs, and aligning your actions with your values. This is the transformative power of Ayurvedic rituals. They nurture the mind, body, and spirit, creating a holistic framework for self-care that resonates with your unique rhythm. These practices empower you to take charge of your well-being, cultivating a sense of autonomy and inner strength.

The potential for transformation lies in the simplicity and consistency of daily Ayurvedic practices. Morning rituals, such as setting intentions or engaging in grounding exercises, lay the foundation for a balanced day. Whether it's a few moments of deep breathing or a gentle yoga sequence, these rituals center you, preparing you to face the day with clarity and focus. As the day winds down, evening rituals invite reflection and relaxation. This might involve a warm bath infused with calming oils or spending time journaling about your experiences and insights. These moments of introspection and relaxation are opportunities to release the day's tensions, fostering a peaceful transition to rest.

Personalizing your Ayurvedic rituals enables you to tailor them to your lifestyle and preferences. Consider incorporating practices that resonate with you, whether it's yoga, meditation, or journaling. You might find that writing in a gratitude journal enhances your sense of peace, or that a few minutes of mindful stretching invigorates your body and mind. Seasonal adjustments also play a crucial role, as Ayurveda encourages aligning with nature's cycles. In the winter, you might cherish warming rituals, such as sipping spiced tea, while summer invites cooling practices, like a refreshing foot soak. Tailoring these rituals to your needs makes them not only more effective but also more enjoyable.

Reflection and self-inquiry become integral aspects of ritual practice, guiding you toward ongoing self-exploration and growth. As you engage in these rituals, consider employing journaling prompts to explore personal intentions. What are you hoping to achieve or understand about yourself? This practice cultivates a habit of self-reflection, prompting you to assess your personal growth and progress regularly. Similarly, reflection exercises can help you gauge how these rituals impact your well-being. Are you feeling more centered, more at peace? This intentional reflection deepens your connection to yourself, illuminating paths to further transformation and joy.

Exploring Your Intentions

Take a few moments each week to explore your intentions in a journal. What goals or aspirations do you have? How can your Ayurvedic rituals support these intentions? Reflect on your progress and any shifts in your mindset or well-being. This practice not only keeps you aligned with your goals but also celebrates your growth along the way.

As this chapter concludes, consider how these rituals can become anchors in your life, grounding you amidst the swirling currents of daily existence. They offer more than just structure; they provide a canvas for self-expression and empowerment. As you embrace these practices, you cultivate a deeper understanding of yourself, paving the way for continued growth and harmony. Next, we will explore how Ayurveda can guide you through life's transitions, supporting you at every stage of life.

Chapter 6: Practical Self-Care Strategies

Imagine waking up to a day filled with endless to-dos, the clock ticking faster than your morning coffee can kick in. Yet, amid this whirlwind, there lies an opportunity to pause, breathe, and care for yourself. This chapter is about incorporating quick and effective Ayurvedic self-care rituals into your daily routine, transforming even the busiest day into a tapestry of peace and rejuvenation.

Finding time for self-care might seem like a luxury in the hustle and bustle of modern life. But what if you could integrate small yet powerful rituals that require just a few minutes? Picture starting your day with a 5-minute Pranayama session. This simple breathwork practice can transform your morning from chaotic to calm. Sit comfortably, close your eyes, and focus on your breath. Inhale deeply through your nose, let the air fill your belly, and exhale slowly. This quick practice centers your mind and energizes your body, setting a positive tone for the day ahead.

As the day progresses and stress begins to creep in, a midday grounding exercise can offer relief. Find a quiet spot, even if it's just for five minutes, and engage in brief meditation or visualization. Close your eyes and imagine yourself in a serene forest, a beach, wherever you feel at peace. Visualize the sights, sounds, and sensations. This practice helps anchor you, offering a mental escape from the day's demands and allowing you to return to your tasks with renewed focus.

Incorporating short, daily rituals can have a profound impact on your well-being. Consider the soothing practice of Abhyanga, or self-massage, using warm sesame oil. Spend just a few minutes massaging your arms, legs, and torso. This ritual nourishes the skin and calms the nervous system, promoting relaxation and a sense of connection with your body. Another simple yet effective practice is an herbal foot soak. Fill a basin with warm water, add Epsom salts and a few drops of lavender oil, and soak your feet for ten minutes. This ritual offers a moment of tranquility, easing tension and grounding your energy.

Consistent self-care practices can lead to significant long-term health improvements, even when brief. Regular rituals improve mood and elevate energy levels, making daily challenges more manageable. These practices enhance focus and productivity, enabling you to approach tasks with clarity and composure. By committing to these small acts of care, you cultivate a foundation of resilience and vitality that supports you through life's ups and downs.

To prioritize self-care in a busy schedule, consider scheduling breaks as you would any important appointment. Set reminders on your phone to pause for a breath or a stretch. Create a self-care toolkit filled with essentials like essential oils, herbal teas, and a cozy blanket. These readily available items make it easier to take a moment for yourself, even on the busiest days. Remember, self-care isn't a luxury; it's a necessity that sustains your well-being and allows you to give your best to the world.

Self-Care Toolkit Checklist

Create a personalized checklist for your self-care toolkit. Include items like a favorite essential oil, a soothing herbal tea blend, and a journal for reflection. Use this checklist as a daily reminder to nurture yourself, ensuring you have the tools you need for moments of peace and renewal.

In embracing these practical self-care strategies, you invite balance and harmony into your life. Each small ritual is a step toward greater well-being, empowering you to navigate life with greater ease and grace.

Ayurvedic Skin Care: Natural Beauty Practices

Imagine waking up each morning, looking in the mirror, and feeling a sense of peace and pride in your skin. This is the essence of Ayurvedic skin care, which emphasizes the use of natural ingredients to nourish and rejuvenate the skin. Ayurveda views skin as a reflection of inner health, emphasizing balance and natural beauty. Emphasizing chemical-free products is crucial. Our skin absorbs what we apply, so choosing natural ingredients over synthetic ones can make a significant difference. Tailoring skincare to your dosha type—Vata, Pitta, or Kapha, ensures that your routine supports your unique skin needs. This personalized approach addresses symptoms and nurtures your skin's essence.

Creating an Ayurvedic skincare routine starts with understanding your skin's nature. If you have Vata skin, characterized by dryness and roughness, opt for hydrating masks with honey and avocado. These ingredients lock in moisture, providing a protective barrier against environmental stressors. Pitta skin, often sensitive and prone to inflammation, benefits from a cooling rose water toner. Rose water soothes irritation and balances the fiery nature of Pitta, leaving the skin calm and refreshed. An exfoliating scrub with chickpea flour can do wonders for Kapha skin, which tends to be oily and congested. This natural cleanser gently removes excess oil and impurities, promoting clarity and balance.

Diet and lifestyle play pivotal roles in skin health, bridging the gap between internal wellness and external beauty. Staying hydrated is essential. Drinking plenty of water flushes out toxins and keeps your skin plump and radiant. Balanced meals, rich in colorful fruits and vegetables, provide vitamins and antioxidants that nourish your skin from within. Stress also impacts your skin's clarity and glow. Managing stress with activities like yoga or meditation can enhance your complexion, as stress reduction promotes hormonal balance and skin vitality.

DIY skincare recipes offer an engaging way to integrate Ayurvedic principles into your beauty routine. Try a turmeric and yogurt face mask for a brightening and anti-inflammatory treatment. This simple blend harnesses turmeric's healing properties and yogurt's lactic acid to exfoliate and rejuvenate. Apply it to your face, let it sit for 15 minutes, and rinse off for a radiant glow. Another luxurious treatment is an almond oil and saffron night serum. Mix a few strands of saffron with almond oil and apply it before bed. Saffron's antioxidants and almond oil's nourishment work together, revitalizing your skin overnight.

Ayurvedic Skincare Routine Checklist

Create a checklist for your personalized Ayurvedic skincare routine. List your chosen products and treatments, aligning them with your dosha type. Use this checklist to guide your daily regimen, ensuring consistency and care.

In Ayurveda, skin care is more than just a routine; it's a way of honoring your body and its connection to nature. By embracing these natural beauty practices, you invite radiance and health into every pore.

Sleep and Ayurveda: Enhancing Restorative Sleep Naturally

In Ayurveda, sleep is not just a part of your daily routine; it's a pillar of health, as crucial as diet and exercise. It restores balance, rejuvenates your spirit, and maintains your vitality. Sleep quality directly connects to the balance of your doshas—Vata, Pitta, and Kapha. Each dosha influences how you sleep, with Kapha's calming nature promoting rest and Vata's energy sometimes causing restlessness. Regular sleep patterns are vital, acting as a stabilizer in your body's rhythmic dance.

To improve sleep quality, Ayurveda suggests embracing an evening wind-down routine. As the sun sets, dim the lights and let your environment mirror the calming glow of twilight. Brew a cup of calming herbal tea, perhaps with chamomile or lavender, and let its warm steam relax your senses. These simple acts prepare your mind and body for rest. Incorporate sleep-inducing herbs like Ashwagandha and Brahmi. Ashwagandha, known for its adaptogenic properties, helps calm the mind and reduce anxiety. Brahmi, a revered herb, enhances mental clarity while promoting a sense of peace. Consider taking these in tea form or as supplements to support a seamless transition into sleep.

Creating a sleep-friendly environment involves nurturing a space that encourages rest. Keep your bedroom cool and dark, mimicking the natural conditions of night. This helps regulate your body temperature, ensuring uninterrupted sleep. Consider soundscapes that soothe, perhaps white noise or the gentle hum of natural sounds, such as rain or a babbling brook. These auditory comforts can help drown out disruptions, allowing your mind to unwind and drift into a deep, restorative sleep.

Your daily habits play a crucial role in sleep health. Reducing caffeine intake, especially in the afternoon, helps prevent the jittery energy that can keep you awake. Opt for herbal teas or decaffeinated options as the day progresses. An evening digital detox is equally essential. Limiting screen time before bed frees your mind from the stimulating effects of blue light and digital distractions. Instead, engage in offline activities like reading a book or gentle stretching to signal to your brain that it's time to wind down.

Imagine your bedroom as a sanctuary, a retreat where tranquility reigns. Making these adjustments transforms your space into a haven of peace. The calming atmosphere enhances your sleep quality and elevates your overall well-being. It's about creating a routine that honors your need for rest, acknowledging that sleep is not a luxury but a necessity. As you implement these practices, you may notice a profound shift in how you sleep and live, with greater energy and clarity greeting you each morning.

Stress Management: Ayurvedic Techniques for Calmness

Stress can feel like an uninvited guest, always lurking in the background, ready to disrupt your peace. Ayurveda offers a holistic approach to managing stress, focusing on achieving calmness through balance and a regular routine. The key lies in understanding your doshas and how they influence your stress response. Vata types, with their quick minds and restless energy, might find themselves overwhelmed easily. For them, grounding practices like warm baths or gentle yoga can be soothing. Pitta types, driven by intensity, may need cooling activities to diffuse their fiery nature. Kapha types, naturally stable, benefit from energizing practices that prevent stagnation. Establishing a routine provides stability, anchoring you amidst life's uncertainties.

Incorporating stress-relief techniques from Ayurveda into your daily life can make a noticeable difference. Breathing exercises, like Nadi Shodhana, can calm the mind and center yourself. This alternate nostril breathing technique balances the brain's hemispheres, promoting focus and tranquility. Visualization techniques, such as guided imagery, serve as mental retreats. Picture yourself in a peaceful place, imagining every detail, from the feel of the breeze to the sounds around you. These practices provide a mental escape, helping you reset and approach challenges with a clear mind.

Diet and herbs also play a significant role in stress management. Adaptogenic herbs like Tulsi and Ashwagandha are renowned for their ability to reduce stress and promote resilience. Tulsi, also known as holy basil, is revered in Ayurveda for its calming properties and its ability to support the immune system. Ashwagandha, an adaptogen, helps the body manage stress, enhancing mental clarity and energy levels. Pair these herbs with stress-relieving foods like almonds and dark chocolate. Almonds provide magnesium, a mineral that supports nervous system health, while dark chocolate contains antioxidants that reduce cortisol levels. Including these in your diet can create a foundation of calmness and well-being.

Making stress management a habit requires intentionality. Set aside time for relaxation, treating it as a non-negotiable part of your day. Schedule daily breaks to pause, breathe, and check in with yourself. Create a stress-reduction toolkit filled with essentials, such as essential oils and calming music. Lavender oil, known for its soothing effects, can be used in a diffuser or applied to your pulse points. Calming music, whether it's gentle piano melodies or nature sounds, can create an atmosphere of tranquility, helping you unwind. By prioritizing these practices, you cultivate a life where calmness is not just an occasional luxury but a daily reality.

Stress Management Reflection Exercise

Consider setting aside a few minutes each evening to reflect on your stress levels and the effectiveness of your stress-management techniques. Keep a journal to note any patterns or triggers and adjust your practices accordingly. This reflection can be a powerful tool for understanding your stress and refining your approach to managing it.

Stress is an inevitable part of life, but with Ayurveda's guidance, it doesn't have to define your experience. By embracing these techniques, you can create a sanctuary of calm within yourself, ready to face whatever comes your way.

Building Resilience: Strengthening Immunity with Ayurveda

In Ayurveda, resilience is intricately linked to the concept of immunity, which is considered the foundation of health. At the heart of this system lies the notion of Ojas, the essence of vitality and the subtle substance believed to be the source of physical strength and mental clarity. When nurtured, Ojas is like an internal reservoir of energy, fortifying your body against illness. Balanced Agni, or digestive fire, is equally critical, as it ensures that nutrients are properly assimilated, transforming food into energy and vitality. Together, Ojas and Agni create a robust immune system, ready to fend off the challenges of daily life.

There are myriad ways to fortify your body's natural defenses through Ayurveda. Herbal allies like Amla, ginger, and turmeric are revered for their immune-boosting properties. Amla, also known as Indian gooseberry, is a powerhouse of vitamin C, providing antioxidant support and enhancing your body's ability to fight off pathogens. Ginger, with its warming properties, aids in digestion and circulation, keeping your internal systems running smoothly. Turmeric, renowned for its anti-inflammatory properties, supports the immune system and promotes overall well-being. Incorporate these herbs into your daily routine, perhaps in a morning tea or as an addition to your meals, to strengthen your immune system. Regular Abhyanga, or oil massage, is another cornerstone of Ayurvedic practice. Using warm oil, such as sesame or coconut, to massage your body can invigorate circulation, enhance lymphatic drainage, and support detoxification, ultimately bolstering your immune health.

Lifestyle and diet are significant players in maintaining a resilient immune system. A nutrient-rich diet abundant in seasonal fruits and vegetables ensures that your body receives the essential vitamins and minerals it needs. Think of vibrant berries in summer or hearty root vegetables in winter as nature's way of aligning your body with the seasons. Regular exercise, whether it's a gentle yoga session or a brisk walk, keeps your body active, promoting circulation and vitality. In tandem with a balanced diet, these practices lay the groundwork for a resilient and robust immune system.

Adapting your practices to seasonal changes is crucial for maintaining immune resilience throughout the year. As the weather shifts, so do your body's needs. In colder months, indulge in warming foods and spices that stoke your digestive fire and keep you cozy. Come spring, cleanse with lighter meals and detoxifying herbs to shed the heaviness of winter. Embrace summer's bounty of hydrating fruits, and as autumn approaches, prepare with grounding foods that will help you transition into the cooler months ahead. Preventive care, such as regular health check-ups, ensures that you're attuned to your body's needs, allowing you to address any imbalances before they manifest into more significant issues.

By embracing these Ayurvedic strategies, you cultivate a life of balance and vitality, where your immune system stands as a testament to the harmony within. This approach is more than just a series of practices; it's about creating a lifestyle where resilience is second nature, woven into the fabric of your everyday existence. As you integrate these principles, you'll discover a newfound connection to your body's wisdom, empowering you to navigate life's challenges with strength and grace.

Ayurvedic Aromatherapy: Using Essential Oils for Healing

Imagine a fragrant garden where each scent holds the power to calm, invigorate, or heal. This is the essence of Ayurvedic aromatherapy, where the power of scent transcends mere fragrance, reaching into the depths of your mind and body. Essential oils provide a simple way to positively impact your mood and health through their potent therapeutic effects. The right scent can lift your spirits, reduce stress, or help you focus, tailored to your individual dosha type for maximum benefit. Vata types might lean towards grounding scents like sandalwood, while Pittas could find solace in cooling aromas like roses. For Kaphas, invigorating scents like eucalyptus can energize and uplift.

Using essential oils effectively begins with understanding their specific health benefits. Lavender, renowned for its calming properties, is ideal for moments when relaxation is needed. A few drops diffused in your living space can transform the atmosphere into a haven of peace. For those times when mental clarity and focus are essential, peppermint is your ally. Its refreshing scent clears the mind and sharpens concentration, making it ideal for study or work environments. Whether you're seeking relaxation or stimulation, there's an essential oil to suit every need.

Emotional well-being is profoundly influenced by aromatherapy. The right blend of oils can shift your mood and ease stress levels. Calming blends, such as chamomile and sandalwood, offer a gentle embrace to frazzled nerves. These oils help soothe tension and promote a sense of peace, making them perfect for unwinding after a long day. On the other hand, energizing blends like eucalyptus and lemon can invigorate your spirit, providing a burst of positivity when you feel sluggish or down. You can alter your emotions by simply inhaling these scents, creating an environment that supports your mental health.

Incorporating aromatherapy into daily routines is both practical and rewarding. Diffusing essential oils creates a calming atmosphere in your home or workspace, subtly transforming the energy around you. You can also make DIY aromatherapy blends tailored to your specific needs. Mix a few drops of your chosen essential oils with a carrier oil, such as almond or jojoba, and apply to pulse points for a personalized fragrance that supports your well-being throughout the day. These small rituals can have a significant impact, offering moments of calm and clarity in a busy world.

As we conclude this chapter on practical self-care strategies, remember that each practice, whether it's aromatherapy or another Ayurvedic technique, provides a path to balance and wellness. These small yet powerful tools are threads in the tapestry of a healthy, harmonious life. In the next chapter, we'll explore how Ayurveda can guide you through life's transitions, lending its wisdom to every stage and challenge. Each step you take in this journey deepens your connection to yourself and the world around you, fostering resilience and vitality.

Chapter 7: Overcoming Common Objections and Misconceptions

Imagine you're standing at the edge of a vast library, where each book offers ancient wisdom and modern insights. Like this library, Ayurveda may seem daunting at first glance, filled with complex terms and practices. Yet, as you open each book, you find stories that resonate, ideas that click, and knowledge that feels like home. If you've ever felt overwhelmed by the complexity of Ayurveda, you are not alone. Many newcomers to this world share a similar sentiment. The beauty of Ayurveda lies in its simplicity and accessibility, waiting to be uncovered by those curious enough to explore.

Demystifying Ayurvedic Complexity: Simple Practices for Beginners

At the heart of Ayurveda are the doshas—Vata, Pitta, and Kapha. Think of them as your body's unique blueprint, guiding how you interact with the world. Vata, the energy of air and space, governs movement and creativity. It's the flutter of a thought, the breeze of inspiration. Pitta, a blend of fire and water, fuels your metabolism and passion. It's the warmth of a hearty laugh or the intensity of focus. Kapha, rooted in earth and water, provides stability and structure, like the comforting embrace of a loved one. Each dosha influences your physical tendencies and emotional patterns, creating a dynamic interplay that makes you, uniquely you.

Stepping into Ayurveda doesn't require a deep dive into complex theories. Instead, begin with foundational practices that are both simple and transformative. Start your morning with tongue scraping, a gentle act that clears toxins collected overnight. Follow with a glass of warm water and a slice of lemon.

This humble ritual awakens your digestive system, setting a harmonious tone for the day ahead. Incorporating these small steps can become a cherished part of your morning routine, offering a moment of mindfulness as you transition into the day.

Ayurveda seamlessly integrates into modern life, offering practices that align with your daily rhythm. Imagine preparing a simple kitchari, a comforting dish of rice and mung beans, spiced with turmeric and cumin. It's a meal that nourishes and balances, easy to prepare even on a busy schedule. Moreover, self-care can easily fit into your routine. Consider taking a five-minute meditation break, a pause to breathe and center your thoughts amidst the hustle. These practices don't demand significant time or effort but provide profound benefits, enhancing your well-being with subtle grace.

As you embrace these practices, remember that Ayurveda is not about perfection. It's about exploration and connection, a journey to understanding your unique needs and rhythms. By starting small and staying curious, you can weave Ayurveda into your life, enriching each day with its timeless wisdom.

Time-Efficient Ayurveda: Integrating Practices into a Busy Schedule

Imagine waking up to a day packed with responsibilities yet finding moments of calm amidst the chaos. Many of us face the misconception that embracing Ayurveda demands hours of dedication and complex routines. However, the truth is that Ayurveda can fit seamlessly into even the busiest of lives. It's all about integrating practices that align with your schedule, creating a rhythm that supports rather than disrupts your daily life. Consider how you can streamline your routines by combining practices. For instance, pair a short meditation session with meal preparation. As you chop vegetables or simmer a pot of soup, take a few moments to breathe deeply and center your thoughts.

This enhances your mindfulness and infuses your cooking with positive energy, making each meal a nourishing experience for body and mind.

Time-efficient Ayurvedic practices are not about grand gestures but about small, meaningful actions. Like a three-minute Pranayama session, quick breathing exercises can offer a powerful reset. Whether you're in the office, at home, or on the go, a few moments of focused breathing can clear your mind and refresh your spirit. This practice is simple yet profound, offering a pause that recharges your energy and enhances your focus. Similarly, consider the benefits of a brief self-massage with aromatic oils before bed. It doesn't have to be elaborate, a few minutes of gentle pressure on your feet or shoulders can alleviate tension and promote restful sleep.

The beauty of Ayurveda lies in its celebration of small, consistent efforts over time. It's the daily practices, however modest, that accumulate to create lasting change. Imagine adding one new Ayurvedic habit each week. Perhaps you start with drinking warm lemon water in the morning, then incorporate a daily five-minute meditation the following week. These incremental changes build a foundation of wellness that's sustainable and impactful. Over time, these small actions become second nature, weaving wellness into the fabric of your life without overwhelming you.

Maintaining consistency amidst a busy life requires setting realistic goals. It's easy to feel motivated initially, but maintaining momentum is where the real challenge lies. Begin with one practice that resonates with you, and let it become a part of your routine before adding another. Utilize technology to your advantage by employing apps that track your progress and send gentle reminders. These digital companions can help keep you accountable, celebrate milestones, and nudge you back on track when life's demands threaten to pull you away from your intentions. Motivation can also come from community support. Share your Ayurvedic journey with friends or join online groups to exchange tips and encouragement. Engaging with others can reinforce your commitment and make the experience more enjoyable.

As you integrate Ayurveda into your life, remember that the goal is balance, not perfection. Life will always be busy, and schedules will ebb and flow, but the peace and vitality that Ayurveda brings are worth the effort. These practices create space for well-being amid everything else, offering a sanctuary of calm and resilience. Embrace the flexibility of Ayurveda, adapting it to your unique needs and lifestyle. With each small step, you're crafting a life that honors your ambitions and well-being, proving that Ayurveda truly fits everyone, even those with the busiest schedules.

Cost-Effective Ayurveda: Affordable Solutions for Every Budget

In a world where wellness trends often come with hefty price tags, it's refreshing to realize that Ayurveda offers a path to health that doesn't require emptying your wallet. Many believe that adopting Ayurvedic practices means investing in expensive treatments or exotic ingredients, but the truth is quite different. Ayurveda embraces simplicity, using what is often already within reach. Your kitchen, for instance, is a goldmine of healing potential. Consider ginger and turmeric, two staples found in most spice racks. These ingredients are not only culinary delights but also potent healers. Ginger aids digestion and reduces inflammation, while turmeric boasts powerful anti-inflammatory properties. A simple tea made from these spices can soothe your system and boost your health without costing much more than a few cents.

DIY treatments bring Ayurveda right to your home. You can create herbal pastes and masks that rival store-bought products with a handful of common ingredients. Try mixing turmeric with yogurt for a face mask that brightens and revitalizes your skin. Or blend chickpea flour with water for a gentle exfoliating paste. These treatments are budget-friendly and customizable to suit your skin's needs. They reflect Ayurveda's ethos of using nature's bounty to nourish and heal.

When considering where to focus your Ayurvedic investments, prioritize quality over quantity. A few key purchases can make a significant impact. High-quality ghee, for instance, serves as a versatile ingredient in cooking and a soothing balm for dry skin. It's a staple in many Ayurvedic recipes, adding richness and aiding digestion. Essential oils also offer a wealth of benefits. Lavender for calming, eucalyptus for clearing, and peppermint for invigorating, all can be used in diffusers, baths, or massages. These oils are small investments with significant returns, enhancing your well-being in multiple ways.

Practicing Ayurveda on a budget involves innovative strategies and resourcefulness. Buying herbs in bulk is one such strategy. Not only does it save money, but it also ensures you have a steady supply of frequently used items like cumin, fennel, and coriander. Community resources can further support your practice without incurring additional costs. Many local health centers and community colleges offer free or low-cost Ayurvedic cooking and wellness classes. These workshops offer valuable knowledge and provide an opportunity to connect with others on a similar path.

One of Ayurveda's most significant benefits is its preventive nature, which can lead to long-term savings. By focusing on maintaining balance and health, Ayurveda reduces the need for costly medical interventions in the long run. Preventive health practices, such as regular detoxification and stress management, can stave off chronic conditions, minimizing future healthcare expenses. Ayurveda's holistic lifestyle enhances physical health and improves mental and emotional well-being. This comprehensive approach often leads to a higher quality of life, where vitality, peace, and happiness are more easily sustained.

Embracing Ayurveda doesn't have to be an expensive endeavor. With creativity and mindfulness, you can incorporate these practices into your life without straining your budget. Simple home remedies, DIY treatments, and thoughtful investments lay the foundation for a wellness that supports you now and for years to come.

Navigating Skepticism: Evidence-Based Benefits of Ayurveda

Skepticism surrounding Ayurveda often stems from a lack of understanding or exposure to its time-honored practices. Many people question its efficacy, perhaps due to its ancient roots and holistic approach, which differ from conventional medicine. Yet, Ayurveda stands on a foundation of evidence-based benefits that have been validated through research and clinical trials. For instance, studies on herbal remedies commonly used in Ayurveda, such as Ashwagandha, have shown promising results. Ashwagandha has been clinically proven to reduce stress and anxiety levels, showcasing its effectiveness beyond anecdotal evidence. Similarly, turmeric, another Ayurvedic staple, has been extensively studied for its anti-inflammatory properties, with research indicating its potential to aid in managing chronic conditions, such as arthritis.

Scientific validation also extends to practices like yoga and meditation, integral components of Ayurveda. Research highlights their positive impact on mental and physical health, including improved flexibility, reduced stress, and enhanced emotional well-being. A study published in the Journal of

Alternative and Complementary Medicine found that regular yoga practice significantly lowers stress levels and improves overall health markers. Meditation has also gained traction in scientific communities for its ability to promote relaxation and focus. These findings underscore how Ayurveda's practices are more than just ancient wisdom; they are validated tools for enhancing modern health.

Real-life examples of Ayurveda's impact further bolster its credibility. Testimonials from individuals who have experienced profound health transformations are abundant. Take, for example, the story of a woman who struggled with chronic digestive issues for years. Conventional treatments brought little relief, but incorporating Ayurvedic dietary practices and herbal supplements led to significant improvements. Her testimony highlights how Ayurveda can offer solutions where other methods may falter, providing a path to wellness that feels both personal and profound.

The integration of Ayurveda into modern healthcare is another testament to its efficacy. Many hospitals and clinics now incorporate Ayurveda into their comprehensive treatment plans. These integrative health clinics recognize the value of combining traditional practices with Western medicine, offering patients a holistic approach to care. For instance, some hospitals have begun incorporating Ayurvedic therapies, such as Panchakarma, a detoxification process, into their treatment offerings, providing patients with additional options for healing. Collaboration between Ayurvedic practitioners and Western medical doctors is becoming increasingly common, resulting in combined treatment plans that address both symptoms and underlying causes. This partnership highlights the potential for Ayurveda to complement conventional medicine, offering a broader spectrum of care.

Numerous resources are available for those interested in exploring Ayurveda's research-backed benefits in more detail.

Ayurvedic journals and publications provide a wealth of peer-reviewed articles, offering insights into the latest studies and findings. Online research databases, such as PubMed, are excellent resources for accessing scientific studies on Ayurveda's practices, ranging from herbal remedies to yoga and meditation. These resources not only enhance the credibility of Ayurveda but also encourage a deeper exploration of its potential. By delving into this research, one can gain a deeper understanding of how Ayurveda continues to thrive in the contemporary world, bridging ancient wisdom with modern science. The synergy between these realms offers a compelling case for Ayurveda as a viable and valuable component of a holistic health approach.

Ayurveda and Western Medicine: Finding a Harmonious Balance

Increasingly, people are accessing healthcare that combines modern medical treatment with Ayurvedic support. These two systems, while different in approach, can work well together. Western medicine is highly effective for diagnosing conditions and managing urgent or complex health issues. Ayurveda, on the other hand, focuses on long-term balance and prevention through diet, lifestyle adjustments, and natural remedies. When used together, they offer a more complete approach to health—addressing immediate symptoms while also supporting the body's overall well-being and underlying imbalances.

The benefits of a holistic approach to healthcare are profound. By integrating both systems, you create a synergy that strengthens the connection between mind and body. Ayurveda encourages you to view health not just as the absence of disease but as a state of complete physical, mental, and emotional well-being. It teaches you to listen to your body's signals and respond with nurturing practices. When combined with Western medicine's precision, this approach offers comprehensive care that considers every aspect of your being. It's about recognizing that healing is multifaceted, requiring attention to the body, mind, and spirit.

Open communication with healthcare providers is crucial for integrating Ayurveda with Western medical treatments. It's important to share your Ayurvedic practices with your doctor, ensuring they understand how these fit into your overall health plan. Begin the conversation by explaining the principles and benefits of Ayurveda, highlighting how it supports your well-being. Provide specific examples of practices you follow, such as dietary choices or herbal supplements, and discuss any potential interactions with prescribed medications. This open dialogue fosters collaboration, allowing your healthcare team to tailor treatments that harmonize with your Ayurvedic lifestyle.

Successful integration stories abound, showcasing the power of combining these two systems. Consider a case where a patient with chronic joint pain found relief through an integrative approach. By complementing conventional treatments with Ayurvedic therapies, such as massage and herbal supplements, the patient experienced enhanced mobility and reduced pain. This example illustrates how Ayurveda can complement Western medicine's effectiveness, providing a broader range of solutions. Institutions like integrative health clinics pave the way for such collaborations, providing patients with access to both Ayurvedic and Western care under one roof. These clinics recognize the value of combining ancient traditions with modern science, creating comprehensive treatment plans that respect the strengths of both systems.

As Ayurveda gains recognition, its integration into mainstream healthcare is likely to increase. This evolution reflects a broader shift toward holistic health, where patients seek solutions that honor their individuality and embrace diverse healing modalities. By exploring this balance, you enhance your health and contribute to a more inclusive and comprehensive healthcare landscape.

In wrapping up this chapter, we've uncovered the synergy between Ayurveda and Western medicine, emphasizing how their integration enriches healthcare. This approach fosters a deeper connection to your health, offering a path that respects and nurtures all aspects of your being. As we move forward, let's explore how Ayurveda can transform daily life, guiding you toward holistic wellness with every step.

Chapter 8: Personal Stories and Transformative Journeys

In the heart of bustling city life, where the pace never seems to relent, many women are caught in a cycle of perpetual exhaustion. Imagine waking up every day feeling drained before the day begins, a sensation that all too many corporate professionals know well. This chapter introduces you to the world of women who, like you, have experienced burnout and found their way back to balance and vitality through the transformative power of Ayurveda. These stories are not just about overcoming challenges but about rediscovering oneself, embracing change, and finding the courage to heal.

From Burnout to Balance: A Journey of Healing and Renewal

Meet Sarah, a corporate professional whose life epitomizes success. Yet, beneath her polished exterior, she battled a silent war with chronic fatigue, insomnia, and anxiety. Her days were a blur of meetings and deadlines, leaving her feeling like a shadow of her former self. Sarah's wake-up call came when her body refused to push any further, forcing her to confront the reality of burnout. She decided it was time to seek a solution beyond the quick fixes she'd grown accustomed to. This was the beginning of her journey toward renewal.

Sarah's initial steps involved embracing the wisdom of Ayurveda, a holistic approach that resonated with her need for a deeper connection to her body and mind. She began by adopting daily routines known as Dinacharya, which introduced rhythm and balance back into her frenetic lifestyle. These practices included rising with the sun to sit quietly in meditation, allowing her mind to find peace before the chaos of the day ensued. Incorporating adaptogenic herbs like Ashwagandha played a crucial role in her recovery, offering stress relief and fostering resilience. Slowly, Sarah returned to a state of vitality she hadn't experienced in years.

The emotional and mental transformation Sarah underwent was profound. Through journaling and self-reflection, she processed the layers of stress and expectation that had accumulated over time. This introspective practice became a tool for emotional healing, enabling her to articulate and release her feelings. As Sarah embraced the principles of Ayurveda, she discovered a newfound mental clarity and emotional stability. The noise in her mind quieted, allowing her to focus on what truly mattered.

Maintaining balance post-recovery became a pivotal aspect of Sarah's journey. She learned the art of setting boundaries, a crucial step in protecting her newfound well-being. This involved prioritizing self-care, ensuring that her needs were met alongside her professional responsibilities. Sarah discovered the importance of work-life balance and the necessity of saying no to commitments that threatened her peace. These strategies safeguarded her health and empowered her to thrive in all aspects of her life.

Balance and Renewal Checklist

Sarah's story illustrates the transformative potential of Ayurveda. For those inspired to embark on a similar journey, consider creating a checklist that includes key practices and strategies for maintaining a balanced approach. This checklist might feature daily routines, stress-relief techniques, and self-care rituals tailored to your unique needs. Use it as a gentle reminder of the small steps you can take daily to nurture yourself and prevent burnout.

This chapter examines the real-life experiences of women who have adopted Ayurveda as a means of healing and renewal.

Their stories remind us that there is hope even in the face of burnout. Through intentional practices and a commitment to self-care, you too can find your way back to balance, embracing a life filled with vitality and purpose.

Overcoming Digestive Struggles

Imagine battling constant discomfort, where every meal becomes a gamble between nourishment and distress. This was the reality for Maya, a young woman who faced the unpredictable tides of Irritable Bowel Syndrome (IBS). Her journey began with persistent bloating and irregular bowel movements that disrupted her life. These symptoms left her feeling trapped in a cycle of uncertainty and anxiety. Desperate for relief, Maya turned to Ayurveda, seeking a path that promised temporary alleviation and genuine healing.

Maya's introduction to Ayurveda marked a turning point. She embraced a tailored Ayurvedic diet designed to ease her digestive woes. Her meal plans focused on simplicity and balance, incorporating easily digestible foods that soothed her Agni, the digestive fire. Maya learned to appreciate the power of spices like cumin, coriander, and fennel, which played a pivotal role in her recovery. These spices, known for their digestive properties, became staples in her kitchen, transforming her meals into healing rituals. As she adopted these dietary changes, Maya noticed a gradual yet profound shift in her digestive health.

Lifestyle adjustments complemented Maya's dietary changes, creating a holistic approach to healing. She introduced mindful eating practices, such as learning to slow down and savor each bite. This practice improved her digestion and helped her reconnect with her body, fostering a sense of gratitude and awareness. Maya's routine began to reflect a new rhythm, one that prioritized her well-being over the rush of daily life. These changes created a foundation of stability, allowing her to experience significant improvements in her digestive health.

Over time, the benefits of Ayurvedic healing extended beyond the physical realm. Maya experienced sustained improvements that transformed her quality of life. Her energy levels soared, leaving her feeling revitalized and capable of tackling each day with vigor. The brain fog that once clouded her thoughts lifted, revealing a newfound mental clarity. This clarity empowered Maya to pursue her passions and interests with renewed enthusiasm, free from the constraints of her previous struggles.

Digestive Health Reflection Exercise

Consider an exercise that encourages reflection on your own digestive health journey. Use a journal to track your symptoms, dietary changes, and lifestyle adjustments. Note any improvements or challenges your encounter, creating a record that helps you understand your body's unique needs. This exercise can be a valuable tool for personal growth and empowerment, guiding you toward a deeper connection with your health.

Through the lens of Ayurveda, Maya's story becomes a testament to the power of holistic healing. Her experience underscores the potential for transformation when one embraces a comprehensive approach that addresses both body and mind. By sharing her journey, we hope to inspire others to explore the possibilities of Ayurveda, encouraging individuals to take charge of their digestive health and find their paths to wellness.

Hormonal Harmony: Personal Triumphs with Ayurveda

During a life transition, many women find themselves grappling with hormonal changes that seem to upend their world. Meet Lisa, a middle-aged woman who faced the challenges of menopause head-on. Her days were marked by intense hot flashes and unpredictable mood swings that left her feeling like a stranger in her skin. These symptoms became constant companions, disrupting her life in ways she hadn't anticipated. Lisa's story is one of resilience and transformation as she turned to Ayurvedic wisdom to navigate this tumultuous phase. Her initial struggles were daunting, yet they became the catalyst for a profound shift toward hormonal harmony.

Lisa's journey began with the introduction of Ayurvedic interventions tailored to her needs. The use of herbal allies, such as Shatavari and Ashoka, became integral to her healing process. Shatavari, often hailed as a woman's best friend in Ayurveda, offered her gentle support for hormonal regulation, easing the emotional rollercoaster she had been riding. Ashoka, known for its cooling properties, helped soothe and stabilize her system. Alongside these herbs, Lisa embraced cooling pranayama techniques. These breathing exercises became her refuge, providing much-needed relief from the intense heat of her hot flashes. Each breath became a step toward balance, a calming force in the storm of change.

As Lisa embraced these practices, she noticed a transformation that extended beyond the physical. The emotional and psychological shifts she experienced were profound. The mood swings that once dictated her days began to subside, replaced by a newfound emotional stability. Lisa found herself more centered, able to approach life's challenges with a clear mind and an open heart. This transformation brought with it an unexpected gift—enhanced self-confidence. As she navigated her way through menopause with grace and resilience, Lisa discovered a newfound sense of empowerment. She embraced life's transitions with newfound vigor, ready to seize each day with open arms.

Sustaining hormonal health became a priority for Lisa, as she sought to maintain the balance she had achieved. Regular health check-ups became a cornerstone of her routine, allowing her to monitor hormonal levels and make informed decisions about her well-being. Lisa committed to continuous lifestyle modifications, understanding that consistency was key. She prioritized exercise, finding joy in activities that energized her body and spirit. A balanced diet rich in nourishing foods provided the foundation for her well-being, supporting her body's natural rhythms. These practices became part of her daily life, ensuring that the harmony she had worked so hard to achieve remained a constant presence.

Hormonal Health Reflection Section

Consider setting aside time for reflection for those inspired by Lisa's story. Use a journal to explore your relationship with hormonal health, documenting changes, challenges, and triumphs. This practice offers a space to connect with your body and emotions, fostering a deeper understanding of your unique journey. You can cultivate awareness and gratitude for the balance you create through reflection.

Embracing Self-Care

Imagine the life of a caregiver named Linda, whose days revolved entirely around others. She was a pillar of strength for her family, yet she forgot to care for herself somewhere along the way. Neglecting her own needs seemed natural, part of the job, until the weight of it became too much to bear. Linda realized she was losing herself in the process of caring for everyone else. The constant demands left her feeling overwhelmed and depleted. It was then that she decided to turn the spotlight inward, to rediscover self-care and its potential for transformation.

Linda's journey into self-care began with the ancient practices of Ayurveda, which offered her a roadmap back to herself. Daily Abhyanga, a self-massage ritual, became her sanctuary. The warm oil on her skin was more than just soothing; it was a moment of connection and self-love. This practice became a ritual that symbolized her commitment to herself, promoting relaxation and mental peace. Alongside this, Linda incorporated regular yoga sessions into her routine. These sessions were not just about physical health; they became a space for her to breathe, to be present, and to find clarity amidst life's chaos. Through these practices, she began to reclaim her time and energy, learning that nurturing herself was not selfish, but essential.

As Linda continued to embrace self-care, she experienced profound emotional growth. She began to recognize her own needs and boundaries, a revelation that empowered her to make choices aligned with her well-being. This newfound self-awareness fostered a deeper understanding of herself, enabling her to communicate her needs with confidence. Linda's journey highlighted the empowering effects of self-care, showing her that she was worthy of the same care she so willingly gave to others. This empowerment was not just a fleeting feeling; it was a transformation that instilled lasting confidence in her ability to navigate life's challenges.

Prioritizing self-care brought long-term benefits that Linda could never have imagined. She established a nurturing routine that became the foundation of her daily life. Simple acts, such as morning meditation or evening reflection, became her anchors, grounding her amid life's unpredictability. Linda also found strength in community, connecting with like-minded individuals who shared her commitment to well-being. This support network encouraged, shared wisdom, and a sense of belonging. Together, they celebrated small victories and supported each other through challenges, reinforcing the importance of self-care as a collective journey.

Self-Care Reflection Journal

Consider setting aside time each week to reflect on your self-care practices. Use a journal to explore your experiences, noting what nourishes you and what feels burdensome. This reflection can help you identify areas where you might want to focus more attention or make adjustments. Over time, this practice can guide you in creating a self-care routine that truly supports your well-being, fostering empowerment and resilience.

Through Linda's narrative, we see the transformative power of embracing self-care. Her story reminds us that taking time for oneself is not a luxury but a necessity. By weaving Ayurveda into her life, Linda discovered a path to empowerment, confidence, and lasting well-being. As you explore your own self-care journey, remember that every step you take towards nurturing yourself is a step towards a more empowered and fulfilling life.

Cultural Connection: Finding Identity through Ayurveda

In a bustling metropolis, where skyscrapers touch the clouds and cultures intertwine, lives a young woman named Priya. As a second-generation immigrant, Priya often felt caught between two worlds. Her parents' traditions seemed distant, like echoes from a life she barely knew, while the fast-paced Western culture pulled her in another direction. Growing up, she felt a disconnect between her heritage and the world she inhabited on a daily basis. But things began to shift when she stumbled upon Ayurveda, an ancient practice deeply rooted in her ancestry. This discovery sparked a curiosity that led her on a path to reconnect with her cultural roots.

Priya's first steps involved immersing herself in the rituals her family had practiced for generations. She was drawn to seasonal celebrations, participating in traditional festivals that she'd once considered outdated. These rituals, rich in symbolism and meaning, resonated deeply with her. She began learning from her family elders, absorbing the wisdom they shared about Ayurvedic practices that had been passed down through generations. With each story and lesson, Priya felt a growing sense of belonging, a connection to her heritage she'd longed for.

As Priya delved deeper into Ayurveda, a transformation began to unfold. She experienced an enhanced cultural pride, embracing her heritage with a newfound passion. The traditions that once felt foreign have now become an integral part of her identity. Engaging with Ayurveda also sparked a spiritual awakening, deepening her connection with both herself and her ancestry. Priya discovered that the practice of Ayurveda wasn't just about health; it was a bridge that connected her past and present, allowing her to honor her roots while thriving in modern society.

Maintaining cultural practices in today's fast-paced world can be challenging, but Priya found ways to integrate tradition with contemporary living. She learned to balance tradition and modernity, blending cultural practices with the demands of everyday life. This meant incorporating Ayurvedic principles into her daily routine, from morning rituals to dietary choices, in an authentic and manageable way. Priya also engaged with cultural communities, participating in events and gatherings celebrating her heritage. These connections provided a sense of community and support, reinforcing her commitment to preserving her cultural identity.

Cultural Reflection and Integration Journal

Take a moment to reflect on your cultural connections. Use a journal to explore your relationship with your heritage, documenting the traditions that resonate with you and how you integrate them into your life. This practice can serve as a meaningful way to connect with your roots and deepen your understanding of your cultural identity.

Through Priya's story, we see how Ayurveda can be a powerful tool for cultural connection and identity formation. Her journey highlights the transformative potential of embracing one's heritage, fostering a sense of pride and belonging. By weaving Ayurveda into her life, Priya discovered a path to personal growth and spiritual fulfillment, honoring her ancestry while embracing the present. Her experience reminds us that our cultural roots are not just a part of our past; they are a vibrant thread woven into the fabric of who we are, guiding us on our path to self-discovery.

Transformative Change: The Path to Holistic Health and Well-being

Imagine waking up every day with a chronic illness, where pain and fatigue paint your reality with a brush of relentless struggle. This was Jessica's life before discovering Ayurveda. Her days were consumed by an exhausting battle against her own body. The simplest tasks seemed Herculean. Yet, within this personal turmoil, a spark of hope appeared when she encountered the Ayurveda holistic system that promised a new beginning. Jessica's path to wellness was not a simple one, but it was transformative. She adopted a comprehensive approach that combined diet, lifestyle, and spiritual practices, resulting in a profound improvement in her overall well-being.

Jessica's integration of Ayurvedic practices began with personalized consultations. These consultations offered tailored treatment plans that addressed her unique constitution and imbalances. Her diet was overhauled to include fresh, organic foods that supported her healing. Meals became a source of nourishment and strength rather than a source of discomfort. Lifestyle changes were equally pivotal. Daily routines, or Dinacharya, provided structure and stability, while spiritual practices like meditation and yoga connected her to a more profound sense of purpose. This multidimensional approach enabled Jessica to address not only the physical symptoms but also the emotional and spiritual aspects of her health.

The impact of these changes was nothing short of remarkable. Physically, Jessica experienced a resurgence of vitality and strength. Activities that once seemed impossible became part of her daily life. Emotionally, she developed resilience and enhanced coping mechanisms. She learned to navigate challenges with grace and poise. Spiritually, she found fulfillment and connection, discovering a sense of peace and purpose she hadn't known before. This all-encompassing change transformed Jessica's view of health, showing her that wellness is not just the absence of illness but a state of complete harmony.

Sustaining this holistic health required continuous self-reflection and adaptation. Jessica understood that health is a dynamic process that evolves in response to her changing needs and circumstances. She committed herself to ongoing learning, exploring new Ayurvedic knowledge and practices to support her journey. This commitment ensured that her health practices remained relevant and practical over time. Jessica's story is a testament to the transformative power of Ayurveda, illustrating that with the right tools and mindset, holistic health is within reach.

As we conclude this chapter, remember that the path to holistic health is a personal and evolving process. The stories shared here demonstrate the potential for profound change when we embrace a comprehensive approach to well-being. Each individual's journey is unique, yet the common thread is the pursuit of balance and harmony in all aspects of life. As we move forward, consider how these principles can be woven into your own life, guiding you toward a state of health and fulfillment that resonates with your true self.

In the next chapter, you'll find simple recipes to support your continued journey toward holistic health and well-being.

Chapter 9: Eat Well, Feel Well: Simple Ayurvedic Recipes

What we eat can either support our balance or throw us further off track. In Ayurveda, food is more than fuel; it's medicine, daily care, and a form of self-respect. This chapter presents simple, nourishing recipes specifically designed for women, with a focus on hormone support, emotional well-being, and digestive ease. You'll find everyday meals, calming drinks, and satisfying snacks that align with your cycle, your dosha, and the seasons. These recipes are flexible, approachable, and created to fit into a busy modern life, because caring for yourself shouldn't be complicated.

Ayurvedic Kitchen Essentials: Stock Your Ayurvedic Pantry

These basic ingredients appear often in Ayurvedic recipes and support digestion, hormones, and immunity:

- Ghee
- Turmeric
- Cumin, coriander, fennel
- Dates and sesame seeds
- Mung dal
- Seasonal fruits and veggies

Recipes:

Cucumber & Dill Cooling Salad

Supports digestion and soothes Pitta dosha

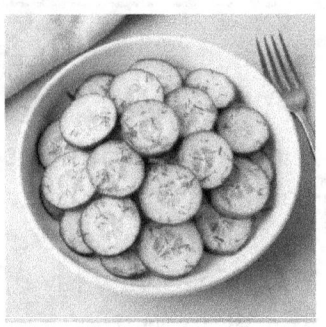

Ingredients (2 servings):
- 1 large cucumber, thinly sliced
- 1 tsp fresh dill (or ½ tsp dried)
- Juice of ½ lemon
- Pinch of rock salt
- Optional: 1 tsp plain yogurt for added creaminess

Instructions:
1. Toss cucumber slices with lemon juice, dill, and salt.
2. Optionally, mix in yogurt for a probiotic boost.
3. Serve chilled or at room temperature.

Spiced Yogurt with Cumin

Combines probiotics with digestive spice

Ingredients (1 serving):

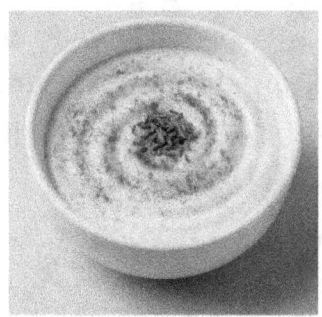

- ½ cup plain yogurt (cow's milk or plant-based)
- ¼ tsp roasted cumin powder
- Pinch of Himalayan salt
- Optional: chopped mint or coriander

Instructions:

1. Mix all ingredients until smooth.
2. Eat as a side dish or digestive snack.

Simple Lentil Digestive Soup

Fiber-rich, warming, and easy to digest

Ingredients (2 servings):

- ½ cup red lentils (masoor dal)
- 3 cups water
- 1 tsp ghee or sesame oil
- ¼ tsp turmeric, ½ tsp cumin
- Pinch of hing (asafoetida), salt to taste
- Optional: spinach or zucchini for added fiber

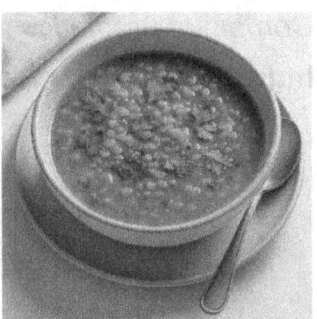

Instructions:

1. Rinse lentils and simmer with turmeric and water until soft (~20 min).
2. In a small pan, heat ghee and toast cumin + hing.
3. Mix into the soup, season, and serve warm

Stewed Apples with Cinnamon

Light and sattvic digestive breakfast or snack

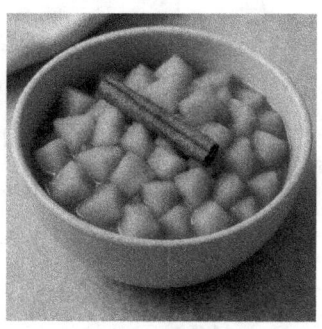

Ingredients (1 serving):
- 1 apple, peeled and chopped
- ¼ tsp cinnamon
- Splash of water
- 1 tsp ghee (optional)

Instructions:
1. Simmer chopped apple with water and cinnamon for 5–7 min.
2. Stir in ghee before serving.

Quinoa with Ginger & Veggies

Light grain bowl for Kapha digestion

Ingredients (2 servings):
- ½ cup quinoa, rinsed
- 1 ¼ cups water
- 1 tsp grated fresh ginger
- 1 small carrot, diced
- ½ zucchini, diced
- 1 tsp olive oil or ghee
- Pinch of salt

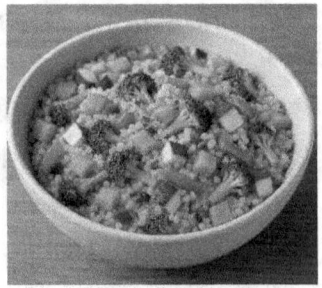

Quinoa with Ginger & Veggies

Instructions:
1. Sauté ginger and veggies in oil for 2–3 minutes.
2. Add quinoa and water; simmer until cooked (~15 min).
3. Fluff and serve warm.

Digestive Herbal Blend Tea (CCFG)

Cumin-Coriander-Fennel-Ginger tea

Ingredients (1–2 servings):
- ½ tsp cumin seeds
- ½ tsp coriander seeds
- ½ tsp fennel seeds
- 3 thin slices fresh ginger
- 2 cups water

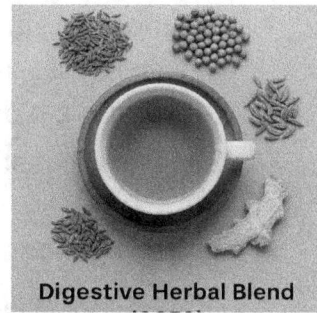
Digestive Herbal Blend

Instructions:
1. Boil all ingredients in water for 7–10 minutes.
2. Strain and sip warm, especially after meals.

Tea & Tonic Recipes

- **Hormone-Balancing Seed Tea:**

  Boil 1 tsp each fennel, coriander, and cumin in water. Strain and sip daily.

  Supports digestion, hormone balance, and reduces bloating.

- **Soothing Rose Petal Tea:**

  Steep dried edible rose petals + cardamom in hot water.

  Great for emotional balance and cooling excess Pitta.

- **Moon Milk for Sleep:**

  Warm plant milk with nutmeg, ashwagandha, and cinnamon.

  Supports deep rest and nervous system regulation.

Warm Spiced Oatmeal (Vata-balancing breakfast)

Ingredients (1 serving):

- ½ cup steel-cut oats
- 1 cup water + ½ cup plant milk
- 1 tbsp ghee (or coconut oil)
- ½ tsp cinnamon + ⅛ tsp cardamom
- Pinch of salt
- 1 tbsp chopped dates or raisins

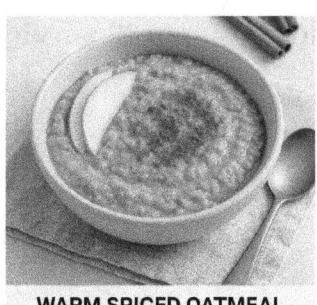

WARM SPICED OATMEAL

Instructions:

1. Bring oats, water, and plant milk to a simmer.
2. Stir in ghee, spices, and salt. Cook for ~10 mins until creamy.
3. Mix in fruit, serve warm.

Dosha tweaks:

- *Pitta*: reduce cinnamon, add a touch of cooling fennel.
- *Kapha*: omit sweet fruit; top with a sprinkle of ginger powder.

Kitchari Power Bowl (Balanced doshas, easy digestion)

Ingredients (2 servings):
- ¼ cup split yellow mung dal
- ⅓ cup basmati rice
- 1 tbsp ghee
- ½ tsp cumin + coriander + turmeric
- Pinch of hing (optional), salt to taste
- 2 cups water + chopped seasonal veggies (e.g., carrot, courgette)

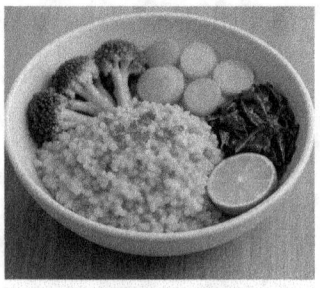

Kitchari Power Bowl

Instructions:
1. Rinse dal + rice. Heat ghee, toast spices briefly.
2. Add grains, water, veggies, salt. Simmer 20–25 mins until soft.
3. Adjust seasoning, garnish with chopped coriander.

Dosha tips:
- *Vata*: add warming ginger.
- *Pitta*: skip hing; use cooling cilantro and lime.
- *Kapha*: reduce ghee, stir in fresh ginger and lemon juice at end

Quinoa & Veggie Power Salad *(Ideal for Kapha-balance)*

Serves 2

Ingredients

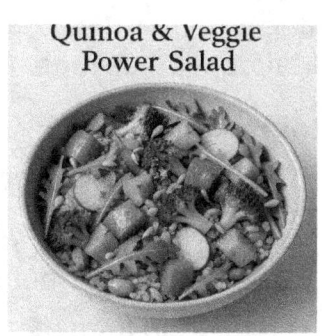

- 1 cup cooked quinoa (cooled)
- ½ cup diced cucumber
- ½ cup grated carro
- 2 spring onions, thinly sliced
- 1 tbsp chopped fresh cilantro
- Dressing: 2 tsp olive or sesame oil, juice of ½ lemon, pinch of cumin, salt & pepper

Method

1. Combine quinoa and veggies in a bowl.
2. Whisk dressing ingredients; pour over salad.
3. Toss gently and serve at room temperature.

Dosha tweaks:

- *Vata*: drizzle extra oil, add a few chopped cashews.
- *Pitta*: swap lemon for cooling mint-infused yogurt drizzle.
- *Kapha*: use minimal oil, add a pinch of black pepper for warmth.

Spiced Sweet Potato & Chickpea Snack *(Balanced afternoon pick-me-up)*

Makes ~4 servings

Ingredients

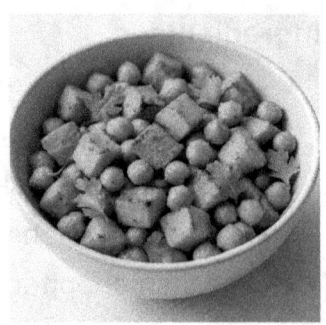

- 2 cups chopped sweet potato
- 1 can chickpeas, drained/rinsed
- 1 tbsp coconut or olive oil
- ½ tsp turmeric, ½ tsp cumin, pinch of salt

Method

1. Toss sweet potato and chickpeas with oil, spices, and salt.
2. Roast at 200 °C (400 °F) for 25–30 min until tender.
3. Serve warm or room temp.

Dosha tweaks:

- *Vata*: add a dash of cinnamon.
- *Pitta*: use olive oil and reduce heat of spices.
- *Kapha*: keep spices bright (extra turmeric) and skip oil.

Warm Cardamom Pear Stew (Evening dessert or snack)

Serves 2

Ingredients

- 2 pears, halved & cored
- 1 tbsp ghee or coconut oil
- 1 tsp cardamom (ground or seeds)
- 1 tbsp raisins or chopped dates
- Splash of water

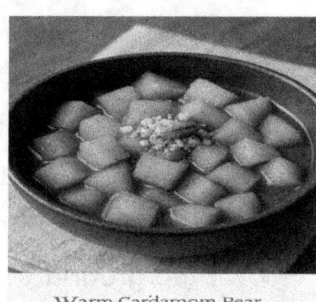
Warm Cardamom Pear

Method

1. Heat ghee, gently cook pears cut-side down for 3 min.
2. Flip, add water, sweetener, cardamom; simmer 5–7 min until soft.
3. Serve warm.

Dosha tweaks:

- *Vata*: add a sprinkle of nutmeg or chopped almonds.
- *Pitta*: use coconut oil and reduce cardamom.
- *Kapha*: add a dash of ginger powder and limit sweetener.

Menstrual Ease Moong-Pear Stew

Gentle and nourishing during menstrual cycles

Ingredients (2 servings)
- 2 ripe pears, halved & cored
- 1 tbsp ghee or coconut oil
- 1 tsp ground cardamom
- 1 tbsp chopped dates or raisins
- Splash of water or plant milk

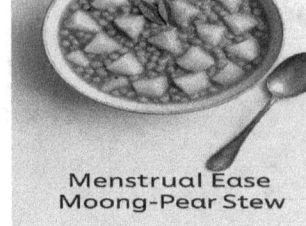

Menstrual Ease Moong-Pear Stew

Instructions
1. Sauté pears cut-side down in oil for 3 min.
2. Flip, add sweetener, cardamom, and water/milk. Simmer 5–7 min.
3. Serve warm—naturally sweet and gentle.

Dosha note: Add nutmeg and nuts for Vata, reduce sweetener for Kapha, use cooling oil (coconut) for Pitta.

Balancing Evening Golden Milk

Recommended nightly ritual

Ingredients (1 cup)

- 1 cup warm almond or oat milk
- ½ tsp turmeric, pinch black pepper
- Pinch cinnamon
- 1 tsp honey or maple syrup (optional)

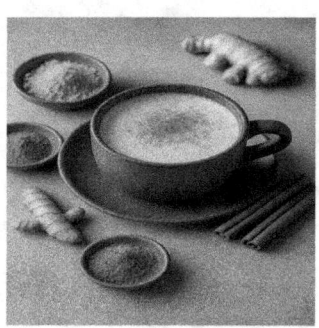

Instructions

1. Warm the milk gently; whisk in spices and sweetener.

Customization: Add ashwagandha for Vata, use lighter milk and omit sweetener for Kapha, reduce spices for Pitta.

Hormone-Balancing Chia & Oat Breakfast Bowl

(Support during menstrual transition)

Ingredients (1 serving)

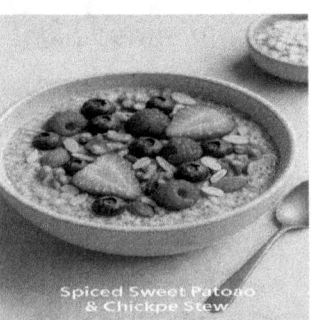
Spiced Sweet Potato & Chickpe Stew

- 3 tbsp rolled oats
- 1 tbsp chia seeds
- ½ tsp ground flaxseed
- ½ tsp cinnamon, pinch of cardamom
- 1 cup warm plant milk
- 1 tsp honey or maple syrup (optional)
- Toppings: sliced berries, nuts, or seeds

Method

1. Warm the milk; stir in oats, chia, flax, and spices.
2. Simmer gently until thickened (~5 min).
3. Sweeten to taste; top with fresh fruit and nuts.

Dosha tips:

- *Vata*: add extra milk and a sprinkle of nutmeg.
- *Pitta*: choose cooling berries; skip sweetener.
- *Kapha*: reduce milk, add ginger, and keep it ligh

PMS Ease Seed Cycling Smoothie

(Perfect for premenstrual & luteal phases)

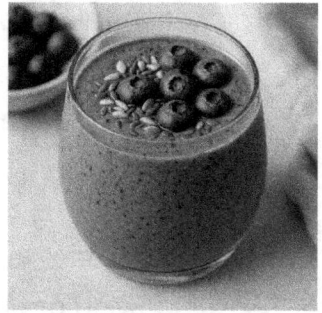

Ingredients (1 serving)
- 1 banana + ½ cup plant milk
- 1 tbsp each: pumpkin & flax seeds (follicular phase), or sunflower & sesame (luteal)
- ½ tsp turmeric + a small piece of fresh ginger
- 1 tsp almond butter or tahini

Method
1. Combine all ingredients in a blender; blend until creamy.
2. Drink mid-morning or as a snack.

Seasonal Spring Mung & Asparagus Khichdi

(For digestion and seasonal cleansing)

Ingredients (2 servings)

- ¼ cup split mung dal + ⅓ cup basmati rice
- 1 tbsp ghee
- ½ tsp cumin, turmeric, coriander
- 1 tsp fresh grated ginger
- 2 cups water + ½ cup chopped asparagus or spring greens
- Salt to taste, garnish with cilantro

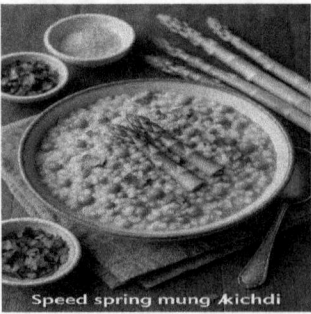
Speed spring mung kichdi

Method

1. Rinse grains; sauté spices in ghee.
2. Add grains, water, ginger, and vegetables.
3. Simmer ~20 min until soft; season and garnish.

Mung dal detoxifies and digests well; asparagus adds springtime vitality

Hormone-Balancing Seed & Date Bars

Great for luteal phase or PMS support

Ingredients (makes 8–10 bars)

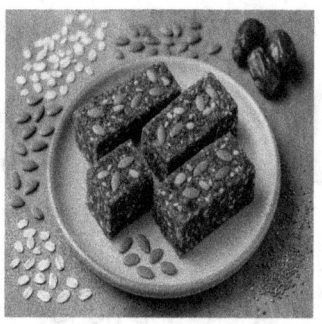

- 1 cup soft Medjool dates, pitted
- ¼ cup sunflower seeds
- ¼ cup sesame seeds
- 2 tbsp ground flaxseeds
- 1 tbsp tahini or almond butter
- ¼ tsp cinnamon
- Pinch of sea salt

Instructions

1. Pulse all ingredients in a food processor until a sticky dough forms.
2. Press the mixture firmly into a parchment-lined container.
3. Chill for at least 1 hour, then slice into bars.
4. Store in the fridge for up to 7 days.

Ideal for the **luteal phase** to help ease PMS and maintain blood sugar stability.

Tridoshic Energy Balls

A dosha-friendly snack to boost mood and focus

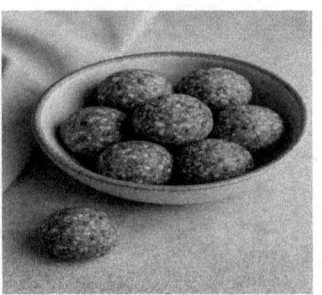

Tridoshic Energy Balls

Ingredients (makes ~12 balls)

- ½ cup rolled oats
- ¼ cup shredded coconut
- ¼ cup almond butter
- 1 tbsp honey or date syrup
- 1 tsp chia seeds
- ½ tsp ground cardamom or cinnamon
- 1–2 tbsp warm water (as needed)

Instructions

1. Mix all ingredients in a bowl. Add water gradually until the mix holds shape.
2. Roll into small balls. Chill for 30 minutes before serving.
3. Store in an airtight container for up to a week.

Calming Ashwagandha-Almond Bites

Helps to reduce stress and support adrenal balance

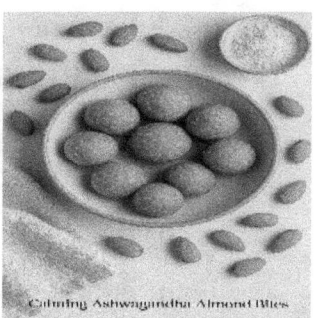

Calming Ashwagandha Almond Bites

Ingredients (makes ~10 balls)

- ½ cup ground almonds (or almond flour)
- 2 tbsp ghee or coconut oil
- 1 tbsp honey or maple syrup
- 1 tsp ashwagandha powder
- ¼ tsp cinnamon
- Pinch of salt

Instructions

1. Mix all ingredients in a bowl until smooth.
2. Roll into balls and chill for 20–30 minutes.
3. Store in the fridge; enjoy 1–2 daily.

Spring (Kapha Season)

Focus: Light, warming, and detoxifying

- **Roasted Chickpeas with Turmeric & Cumin**
  Sprinkle chickpeas with spices and bake until crisp.
- **Steamed Asparagus with Lemon & Black Pepper**
  Helps stimulate digestion and supports liver function.
- **Warm Pear with Ginger & Cinnamon**
  Light and gently sweet, perfect for Kapha balance.

Summer (Pitta Season)

Focus: Cooling, hydrating, and calming

- **Coconut Yogurt with Chia Seeds and Mint**
  Soothes inflammation and supports gut health.
- **Watermelon & Cucumber Salad with Lime**
  Light and cooling, supports hydration and skin clarity.
- **Rice Cakes with Tahini & Date Paste**
  Keeps blood sugar stable without overheating the system.

Autumn (Early Vata Season)

Focus: Grounding, moistening, and warming

- **Date & Oat Muffins with Ghee**
  Supports elimination and energy, ideal for dry skin and digestion.
- **Stewed Apple with Clove & Cardamom**
  Balances Vata and helps regulate morning elimination.
- **Almond Butter on Warm Toasted Rye Crackers**
  Comforting and stabilizing for fluctuating moods.

Winter (Deep Vata Season)

Focus: Heavier, warming, and nourishing

- **Sesame Ladoo (Sesame Balls with Jaggery)**
  Strengthens bones and supports menstrual health.
- **Golden Milk with Ashwagandha & Nutmeg**
  Calms the nervous system and promotes deep sleep.
- **Walnut & Fig Energy Bites**
  Helps with brain fog and low energy, rich in omega-3s.

Snack Planning by Dosha or Cycle Phase

Goal / Phase	Best Snack Type	Example
Vata (irregular, anxious)	Warm, oily, grounding	Almond-date bites, warm pear stew
Pitta (irritable, hot)	Cooling, mildly sweet, light	Chia-mint coconut yogurt, cucumber salad
Kapha (sluggish, heavy)	Light, dry, spicy	Roasted chickpeas, citrus fruit
Follicular Phase	Energizing, protein-rich	Seed cycling smoothie, energy balls
Luteal / PMS Phase	Hormone-supportive, calming	Sunflower bars, calming golden milk
Menstrual Phase	Iron-rich, easy to digest	Stewed apples, sesame ladoo

We'd Love Your Review — Help Others Discover Ayurveda for Her

Thank you for reading *Ayurveda for Her*. I hope the tools, reflections, and recipes in this book have helped you feel more balanced, nourished, and in tune with your body, whether it was a small change in your daily routine or a deeper shift in how you care for yourself, your experience matters.

If this book helped you in any way, I'd be truly grateful if you could take a moment to leave a review. Your words don't just support my work; they help others decide if this book is right for them. Many women are seeking simple, natural ways to improve their well-being. By sharing your honest feedback, you're making it easier for them to find a resource that could truly make a difference in their lives.

Just **click the link or scan the QR code** to leave your review. It only takes a minute, but it can guide someone else toward healing and self-care.

Thank you again for being part of this journey. Your voice can inspire and empower others to take their own steps toward wellness.

https://www.amazon.com/review/create-review/?ie=UTF8&channel=glance-detail&asin=B0FGDLSVXP

Conclusion

As we reach the end of our journey together, let's take a moment to reflect on the core themes we've explored. This book has been about empowering you, the modern woman, to harness the timeless wisdom of Ayurveda. We've explored practical solutions to enhance your digestive health, balance your hormones, and foster holistic well-being, all without the burden of guilt. The knowledge shared within these pages is intended to be a companion, guiding you toward a life where health and harmony are not just goals, but daily realities.

Throughout our exploration, we've emphasized the transformative power of integrating Ayurveda into your life. Understanding your unique dosha is like discovering a personal roadmap to health. Embracing natural remedies and adopting mindfulness practices aren't just about addressing symptoms; they're pathways to profound improvements in your well-being. The small changes you make can lead to significant shifts, leaving you with a vibrant body and a calm and focused mind.

One of the most beautiful aspects of Ayurveda is its emphasis on personalization. Each of us is unique, and our health practices should reflect that. Tailoring Ayurvedic principles to your needs and life stages is crucial. Whether you're a young adult finding your way, a mother nurturing new life, or a woman navigating the changes of menopause, Ayurveda offers tools that can be adapted to suit your journey. Use the insights you've gained to craft a personalized approach that resonates with your body's rhythm and the demands of your life.

While this book provides a foundation, the journey doesn't stop here. Please continue exploring Ayurveda beyond these pages. Engage with local Ayurvedic communities, attend workshops, or consult with practitioners to deepen your understanding of Ayurveda. Ayurveda is a living tradition, rich with opportunities for learning and growth. Dive deeper into its practices and philosophies and discover new ways to enrich your life.

As you stand on the threshold of this new path, I invite you to take actionable steps toward embracing Ayurveda. Start small, perhaps with a morning ritual or a dietary change, and gradually integrate new practices. Pay attention to how these shifts impact your overall health and lifestyle. Notice the moments of clarity, the bursts of energy, and the sense of balance that emerges when you align with nature's wisdom.

In this journey, you're not alone. I encourage you to share your experiences and connect with others who are also exploring Ayurveda. Build a supportive community where you can exchange insights, share successes and setbacks, and grow together. This collective wisdom can be a powerful source of inspiration and encouragement.

Thank you for the trust and engagement you've shown throughout this book. Your commitment to your health and well-being is commendable, and I'm honored to have been a part of your journey. Remember, Ayurveda is not about perfection but about progress and connection. It's about nurturing yourself with compassion and curiosity.

As you close this book, carry with you an uplifting message of empowerment and transformation. Let the principles of Ayurveda inspire you to prioritize your health and embrace the fullness of life. May you find strength in your journey, joy in your discoveries, and peace in your being. Here's to a vibrant, balanced, and fulfilling life, one where you thrive with every breath, step, and moment.

References

- *The doshas explained*
  https://www.keralaayurveda.us/courses/blog/the-doshas-explained/

- *Ayurvedic Care for Women at Any Age*
  https://mapi.com/blogs/articles/ayurvedic-care-for-women-at-any-age?srsltid=AfmBOoo0o6uIto2z0-DWGCDbPxh8s-CF0LZp69mO18jlc6t6A2J-WFLb

- *CONCEPT OF AGNI AND AMA IN AYURVEDA*
  https://www.wjpmr.com/download/article/100082022/1661853345.pdf

- *Dincharya in Ayurveda | Ayurvedic Daily Routine*
  https://www.dabur.com/blog/ayurvedic-daily-routine/dinacharya

- *Menstrual health: An Ayurvedic perspective*
  https://www.herbalreality.com/condition/menstrual-health-ayurvedic-perspective/

- *Navigating Hormonal Acne with Ayurvedic Management*
  https://samwarthika.com/articles/navigating-hormonal-acne-with-ayurvedic-management-holistic-approaches-for-clearer-skin/

- *Ayurvedic Approach to Menopause - Ayurveda*
  https://ayutherapy.com/news/ayurvedic-menopause-management/

- *Can Ayurvedic Medicine Effectively Treat Thyroid Disorders?* https://www.healthline.com/health/ayurvedic-medicine-for-thyroid

- *12 Powerful Ayurvedic Herbs and Spices with Health Benefits* https://www.healthline.com/nutrition/ayurvedic-herbs

- *What Is the Ayurvedic Diet? Benefits, Downsides, and More* https://www.healthline.com/nutrition/ayurvedic-diet

- *Ayurvedic Guidelines for Healthy Eating: Allow 3 Hours or ...* https://www.ayurvedacollege.com/blog/ayurvedic-guidelines-healthy-eating-allow-three-hours-or-more-between-meals/#:~:text=It%20is%20important%20to%20allow,returns%20leads%20to%20poor%20digestion.

- *Sattvic Diet Review: What It Is, Food Lists, and Menu* https://www.healthline.com/nutrition/sattvic-diet-review

- *Ayurveda for Pregnancy and Childbirth* https://www.banyanbotanicals.com/blogs/wellness/tagged/category-pregnancy?srsltid=AfmBOooBZ53UOxrLPkoiHbETqi2pCnbpMiA9EwVR9qmgmWS1pWpJ3Yls

- *Birthing Ayurveda: Postpartum Part 1—Nurturing the Mother* https://www.banyanbotanicals.com/blogs/wellness/birthing-ayurveda-postpartum-nurturing-the-mother?srsltid=AfmBOooXBfjzCZGf4S9mlLgQQGAc9dqgcLrcNXUXmnYt11DIVxgUC2tm

- *Ayurvedic Approach to Menopause - Ayutherapy* https://ayutherapy.com/news/ayurvedic-menopause-management/

- *Ayurvedic Path to Osteoporosis Management Without ...* https://www.pravaayu.com/blog/osteoporosis

- *Meditation in Yoga and Ayurveda* https://www.vedanet.com/meditation-in-yoga-and-ayurveda/

- *Chakra System and their connection with feminine energy* https://certified-excellence.com/topics/2-1-chakra-system-and-their-connection-with-feminine-energy/

- *Pranayama Benefits for Physical and Emotional Health* https://www.healthline.com/health/pranayama-benefits

- *Cultural Competence in Ayurvedic Practices* https://www.awebofwellness.com/blogs/news/cultural-competence-in-ayurvedic-practices?srsltid=AfmBOoqC0gfSUx5MpElqZGjwvkIRCreI3t7sOx4eNTiC50jyBS34E9cG

- *3 Quick Ayurvedic Self-Care Tips for Busy Mornings* https://theskinmixology.com/blogs/wellness-guide/3-quick-ayurvedic-inspired-self-care-hacks-for-busy-mornings

- *A Guide to Ayurvedic Skin Care: Treatments and Products ...* https://www.healthline.com/health/beauty-skin-care/ayurvedic-skin-care

- *A Guide to Sleep Based on Your Ayurvedic Type* https://www.healthline.com/health/sleep/an-ayurvedic-guide-to-sleep

- *Ayurvedic Tips for Stress Management* https://www.dabur.com/blog/health-guides/ayurvedic-tips-stress-management

- *Ayurveda 101: A Beginner's Guide* https://www.thenueco.com/blogs/journal/ayurveda-101-a-beginners-guide?srsltid=AfmBOooPXKTa6VeQwEN_8o9aSAAwMl VVcinwkLUeO4r9Ed0Vj6MVzHBw

- *Ayurveda and Cycles of Time: How the Doshas Rule the Day* https://www.ayurvedacollege.com/blog/ayurveda-and-cycles-time-how-doshas-rule-day/

- *Ayurveda on a Budget: Simple and Affordable Wellness ...* https://eliteayurveda.com/blog/ayurveda-on-a-budget-simple-and-affordable-wellness-routines/

- *Ayurveda Information | Mount Sinai - New York* https://www.mountsinai.org/health-library/treatment/ayurveda

- *How Ayurveda Helped Me Recover from Corporate Burnout in ...* https://girlsguidetolivingabroad.substack.com/p/burnout-to-ayurvedic-consultant-on-koh-phangan

- *Improve Gut Health and Digestion with Ayurveda* https://www.banyanbotanicals.com/pages/ayurvedic-digestion?srsltid=AfmBOoq-0CvzshLi1w_N28Kk80bnet-bIJe4JEmwpT0qyCkquCQfKZnk

- *8 Ayurvedic practices for hormonal harmony* https://theayurvedicclinic.com/8-ayurvedic-practices-for-hormonal-harmony/

- *Traditions, rituals and science of Ayurveda - PMC* https://pmc.ncbi.nlm.nih.gov/articles/PMC4204279/

www.ingramcontent.com/pod-product-compliance
Lightning Source LLC
Chambersburg PA
CBHW052053070526
44584CB00017B/2154